Get Through
First FRCR: MCQs for the Physics Module

Grant Mair BSc (Hons) MB ChB MRCS
Andrew Baird MB ChB MRCS
Andrew Nisbet MB BCh

All Specialty Trainees in Radiology, South East Scotland Programme, The Royal Infirmary of Edinburgh, UK

Consulting Editor

Jerry Williams BA MSc FIPEM

Consultant Medical Physicist, RPA and Head of Radiology Physics Training Programme for South East Scotland, The Royal Infirmary of Edinburgh, UK

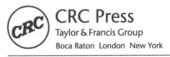

CRC Press
Taylor & Francis Group
Boca Raton London New York

CRC Press is an imprint of the
Taylor & Francis Group, an **informa** business

CRC Press
Taylor & Francis Group
6000 Broken Sound Parkway NW, Suite 300
Boca Raton, FL 33487-2742

© 2010 by Taylor & Francis Group, LLC
CRC Press is an imprint of Taylor & Francis Group, an Informa business

No claim to original U.S. Government works

Visit the Taylor & Francis Web site at
http://www.taylorandfrancis.com

and the CRC Press Web site at
http://www.crcpress.com

Contents

To our families

Preface

To keep pace with technological advances in the workplace and evolving legislation, and as a means of examining all radiological basic science in one sitting, the Royal College of Radiologists (RCR) recently expanded and updated the syllabus for the Part 1 FRCR Physics exam. From March 2009, Part 1 candidates are now examined in all areas of medical physics relevant to radiology. Most notably, the syllabus once again includes ultrasound and magnetic resonance imaging (MRI). In addition, the new exam reflects the continued uptake of digital imaging systems in many departments around the world. From March 2010, a second module in Radiological Anatomy will also be examined in parallel to the Physics module. This book deals only with the Physics module.

All information relating to the exam can be found on the RCR website. The current format is of 40 stems each with 5 subheadings, giving a total of 200 questions. Answers are either 'True' or 'False'; there is no penalty for an incorrect answer so all questions should be attempted. As a candidate you have 2 hours in which to complete the exam. Postgraduate exams can be daunting and while structuring your individual study preparation is a personal choice there is no doubt that answering practice MCQs in parallel with traditional revision techniques will enhance your likelihood of success.

The questions in this book are arranged in a similar format to the exam and we have carefully tried to cover the entire syllabus. Our questions are designed as aids to the revision process, with each question intended to supply a learning point and each chapter to highlight the areas of knowledge required. By working through each chapter we hope you will gain confidence in your knowledge of the key topics as well as identify areas that may require further study. Full answers are given to all the questions, and while they are not intended to be complete descriptions of a subject they should form the basis of further revision. Given the complexity of the subjects covered in this book we accept there will inevitably be some debate or disagreement over our answers. We hope this will stimulate discussion around the subject and may ultimately enhance understanding. To provide additional feedback, each group of questions is assigned a difficulty level, ranging from * (easiest) to ***** (most difficult).

The included mock exam should be attempted under exam conditions and is more representative of the level of difficulty likely to be encountered. Allow 2 hours for completion and score +1 for each correct answer and 0 for incorrect answers. The content of the mock exam is representative of our own experience; it should be noted, however, that the College may choose to examine candidates on any aspect of the curriculum.

The authors are all Specialty Registrars on the South East Scotland Radiology Training Scheme and have all contributed equally to the writing of this book. All were successful in passing the new FRCR Part 1 examination at their first sitting. Jerry Williams is the Head of the Radiology Physics Training Programme for South East Scotland. In addition he is the co-author of *Farr's Physics for Medical Imaging*. We are indebted to him for his guidance and help with the writing of this book. Special thanks also go to Nick Weir, a medical physicist based in Edinburgh, for his help with the MRI chapter.

Finally, we wish you the best of luck and every success in the exam!

Andrew Nisbet
Andrew Baird
Grant Mair

Reference

Allisy-Roberts PJ, Williams J. *Farr's Physics for Medical Imaging*, 2nd edn. Philadelphia: Elsevier, 2008.

Recommended Reading

Allisy-Roberts PJ, Williams J. *Farr's Physics for Medical Imaging*, 2nd edn. Philadelphia: Elsevier, 2007.

Campus Medica. *e-MRI, Magnetic Resonance Imaging physics and technique course on the web.* www.e-mri.org.

Hendee WR, Ritenour ER. *Medical Imaging Physics*, 4th edn. New York: Wiley-Liss, 2002.

Kalender W. *Computed Tomography: Fundamentals, System Technology, Image Quality, Application*, 2nd edn. Weinheim: Wiley-VCH, 2004.

McRobbie DW, Moore EA, Graves MJ, Prince MR. *MRI From Picture to Proton*, 2nd edn. Cambridge: Cambridge University Press, 2007.

Westbrook C, Roth CK, Talbot J. *MRI at a Glance*. Oxford: WileyBlackwell, 2002.

Abbreviations

2D	two-dimensional
3D	three-dimensional
AC	alternating current
ACOP	Approved Code of Practice
ALARP	as low as is reasonably practicable
AP	anteroposterior
ARSAC	Administration of Radioactive Substances Advisory Committee
BMUS	British Medical Ultrasound Society
Bq	becquerel
c	speed of light
Ca	calcium
CCD	charge coupled device
CR	computed radiography
CSF	cerebrospinal fluid
CsI	caesium iodide
CT	computed tomography
CTDI	Computed Tomography Dose Index
CT KUB	computed tomography kidneys, ureters and bladder
CXR	chest X-ray
DAP	dose area product
dB	decibels
DC	direct current
DDI	detector dose indicator
DICOM	Digital Imaging and COmmunications in Medicine
DLP	dose length product
DMSA	dimercaptosuccinic acid
DNA	deoxyribonucleic acid
DQE	detective quantum efficiency
DR	digital radiography
DRL	diagnostic reference level
DSA	digital subtraction angiography
E	energy
e^-	electron
ECG	electrocardiogram
eGFR	estimated glomerular filtration rate
EPI	echo-planar imaging
eV	electron volt (often prefixed with kilo, e.g. keV)
F	fluorine
f	frequency
FDG	fluorodeoxyglucose
FID	free induction decay
FLAIR	FLuid Attenuated Inversion Recovery
FOV	field of view
fps	frames per second
FRCR	Fellow of the Royal College of Radiologists
FSE	fast (turbo) spin echo
GB	gigabyte

GRE	gradient recalled echo
Gy	gray
h	Planck's constant
HSWA	Health and Safety at Work Act 1974
HVL	half-value layer
HSE	Health and Safety Executive
HU	Hounsfield unit
Hz	hertz
I	iodine
ICNIRP	International Commission on Non-Ionizing Radiation Protection
ICRP	International Commission on Radiological Protection
IR(ME)R	Ionising Radiation (Medical Exposure) Regulations
IRR99	Ionising Radiations Regulations 1999
IVU	intravenous urography
J	joule
K_α	alpha characteristic radiation
K_β	beta characteristic radiation
keV	kiloelectron volt
kV	kilovolt
kVp	the peak kilovoltage of an X-ray tube
LET	linear energy transfer
LMP	last menstrual period
lp/mm	line pairs per millimetre
LSF	line spread function
m	mass
mA	milliamperes
MAG3	mercaptoacetyl triglycine
MARS	Medicines (Administration of Radioactive Substances) Regulations 1978
mAs	milliampere-seconds
MB	megabyte
MBq	megabecquerel
MeV	millielectron volt
MDCT	multidetector computed tomography
mGy	milligray
MHRA	Medicines and Healthcare products Regulatory Agency
MI	Mechanical Index
MIBI	2-methoxy isobutyl isonitrile
MinIP	minimum intensity projection
MIP	maximum intensity projection
Mo	molybdenum
MPR	multi-planar reconstruction
MR	magnetic resonance
MRI	magnetic resonance imaging
MTF	modulation transfer function
ms^{-1}	metres per second
mSv	millisievert
m_{xy}	magnetic vector in the x,y-axis

m_z	magnetic vector in the z-axis
N	neutron
NaI	sodium iodide
OD	optical density
OSL	optically stimulated luminescence
P	proton
PA	posteroanterior
PACS	Picture Archiving and Communications System
Pb	lead
PD	proton density
PET	positron emission tomography
PHA	pulse height analyser
PRF	pulse repetition frequency
PVDF	polyvinylidine difluoride
PZT	lead zirconate titanate
QA	quality assurance
RBE	relative biological effectiveness
RF	radiofrequency
Rh	rhodium
RPA	radiation protection advisor
RPS	radiation protection supervisor
RSA	Radioactive Substances Act 1993
SAR	specific absorption ratio
SE	spin echo
SI	Système International
SNR	signal to noise ratio
SPECT	single photon emission computed tomography
SMPTE	Society of Motion Picture and Television Engineers
STIR	short tau inversion recovery
Sv	sievert
T	tesla
Tc-99m	^{99}Technetium metastable
TE	time to echo
TGC	time gain compensation
TI	Thermal Index
TFT	thin film transistor
TLD	thermoluminescent dosimetry
TR	time to repeat
W	tungsten
Xe	xenon
Z	atomic number
z	acoustic impedance
μ	linear attenuation coefficient
β^+	positron

1. For atomic structure:
   a. The atomic number is the number of protons plus electrons
   b. Electrons exist in shells of energy levels around the nucleus
   c. All electrons exist at the same energy level for a given element
   d. A nucleon is smaller than a nucleus
   e. The nucleus of an atom has a net positive charge

2. Elements useful to radiology:
   a. The atomic number of tungsten (W) is 82
   b. The K-edge of barium is approximately 37 keV
   c. The K-edge of calcium (Ca) is approximately 20 keV
   d. The gamma emission of ^{99}Technectium metastable (Tc-99m) is approximately 140 keV
   e. The atomic number of iodine is 53

3. Regarding electromagnetic radiation:
   a. Radio-waves are a form of electromagnetic radiation
   b. Radio-waves travel at 3×8^{10} ms^{-1} in vacuo
   c. X-rays and gamma rays vary only in their origin
   d. Frequency and wavelength are directly proportional to one another
   e. Radio-waves travel in divergent straight lines

4. In the production of X-rays:
   a. Bremsstrahlung refers to the energy gained by electrons as they are accelerated towards the target
   b. Thermionic emission occurs in the target
   c. Bremsstrahlung radiation is formed at the cathode of an X-ray tube
   d. Characteristic radiation is formed at the anode of an X-ray tube
   e. Only about 50% of the energy of the bombarding electrons is emitted as useful X-ray radiation

5. X-ray attenuation:
   a. Is the process where photons are absorbed or scattered thus reducing the photons in the emerging beam
   b. In a monoenergetic beam, the half-value layer increases with depth due to hardening of the beam
   c. Monoenergetic beams are used in digital radiography
   d. The linear attenuation coefficient is inversely proportional to the half-value layer (HVL)
   e. The number of photons in the emerging beam reaches zero after five HVLs

I. Basic Physics: Questions

6. **Attenuation of X-rays:**
   a. In clinical practice, the first and second HVLs are equal
   b. The mass attenuation coefficient of a material decreases with atomic number
   c. Elastic scatter greatly affects the images produced using X-rays
   d. The photoelectric effect leads to complete absorption of X-ray photon energy
   e. The photoelectric effect predominates when diagnostic X-rays meet contrast media such as barium

7. **Regarding an X-ray beam used in clinical practice:**
   a. If the characteristic radiation was removed from a beam the intensity of that beam would increase
   b. The intensity of a beam would diminish by 16 times if you moved from 1 m to 4 m from the source
   c. The inverse square law assumes no absorption or scattering in the medium
   d. The mean energy of the beam is approximately 50% of the operating tube kV
   e. It has a constant HVL

8. **Regarding the Compton effect:**
   a. The Compton effect describes scatter of photons by the tissue
   b. A photoelectron is ejected in a collision with a photon
   c. The free electrons described in Compton scatter are often bound within the valence shell of atoms
   d. The probability of the Compton effect is proportional to the atomic number (Z) cubed
   e. The mass attenuation coefficient for the Compton effect for bone is twice that of soft tissue

9. **Photoelectric effect:**
   a. The photoelectric effect occurs at a maximum when the incident photon energy is just less than the K-edge
   b. Characteristic radiation may be emitted after the photoelectric effect
   c. Most biological damage is caused directly by the ionization of the atom by X-ray photons
   d. At higher energies the photoelectric effect becomes a more common interaction
   e. The photoelectron has energy equal to the energy of the incident photon plus the binding energy of the electron

2

10. **X-ray interactions with matter:**
    a. The photoelectric effect predominates in high kV techniques such as computed tomography (CT)
    b. At 30 keV or less the Compton effect predominates
    c. In diagnostic high kV techniques such as CT pair production becomes a significant effect
    d. In Compton scatter the electron never travels in the backward direction
    e. The probability of Compton scatter occurring is related to the electron density of the material

11. **Regarding luminescence:**
    a. The outermost filled electron band in a luminescent material is known as the conduction band
    b. The process of luminescence is possible only in substances which are manufactured entirely free from impurities
    c. In radiographic detectors the intensity of light emitted from a phosphor is directly proportional to the intensity of energy absorbed from the X-rays or gamma rays
    d. In computed radiography (CR) image processing, the exposed detector plate is heated in order to stimulate the release of light
    e. In personal dosimetry systems, optical stimulated luminescent dosimeters allow a greater sensitivity of measurement compared with thermoluminescent detectors

12. **Radiation:**
    a. Bremsstrahlung radiation can occur at any energy from just above 0 keV to the peak voltage potential in the X-ray tube
    b. K_α radiation describes the emission of a particle of two protons and two neutrons
    c. Characteristic radiation results in specific energy photons being emitted relating to the electron binding energies
    d. Characteristic radiation from the L-shell of tungsten is used in high kV techniques
    e. Beta radiation is commonly used in nuclear diagnostic imaging.

I. Basic Physics: Answers

Ia. False **
Atomic number is the number in the periodic table, defined by the number of protons. Atomic mass number is the number of protons plus the number of neutrons.

Ib. True
Electrons exist at different energy levels described as shells of decreasing energy.

Ic. False
It will take the same amount of energy to dislodge a K-shell electron for different atoms of the same element, but the K-shell electrons and L-shell electrons within the same atom will have different energy levels.

Id. False
Examples of nucleons are protons and neutrons. A nucleus is all the protons plus neutrons of one atom. In hydrogen the single proton is the only nucleon, and thus the nucleon and the nucleus would be the same size.

Ie. True
The nucleus comprises positive protons and neutral neutrons. Negative electrons exist outside the nucleus.

2a. False *
Lead (Pb) has an atomic number of 82. Tungsten (W) has an atomic number of 74.

2b. True
The K-edge of barium is high enough that the photoelectric effect predominates in barium screening.

2c. False
The K-edge of Ca is 4 keV. Common elements in the body have a low K-edge which is why the Compton effect predominates at the higher end of the diagnostic energy range.

2d. True
This is much higher than diagnostic X-ray energies.

2e. True
With a higher atomic number than soft tissue, the K-edge of iodine is also higher. The photoelectric effect therefore predominates at diagnostic X-ray energies; this makes it suitable as a contrast agent.

3a. True *
Radio-waves are the least energetic form of electromagnetic radiation.

3b. False
They travel at $3 \times 10^8 \, \text{ms}^{-1}$ in vacuo.

3c. True
X-rays arise primarily through changes in electron energy state; gamma rays arise from radioactive decay.

3d. False
They are indirectly proportional.

3e. True
This is one of the particle-like properties of electromagnetic radiation.

4a. False ***
Bremsstrahlung can be translated as 'braking' energy, referring to the slowing of the bombarding electron. The electron is slowed by its passage close to the nucleus and gives off the reduction in kinetic energy as electromagnetic radiation.

4b. False
Thermionic emission occurs in the filament of the cathode. This is the method by which electrons are emitted for acceleration to the target.

4c. False
Electrons are produced at the negative cathode and accelerate towards the positive anode, where they can react with the target atoms to produce X-rays.

4d. True
When the electrons hit atoms in the anode they can produce X-rays either through the Bremsstrahlung process or can knock a K-shell electron out of its orbit thus allowing an L- or M-shell electron to drop down and produce characteristic radiation.

4e. False
Typically less than 1% of the energy is converted to useful X-ray radiation.

5a. True **
This occurs to a greater or lesser extent in different tissues; it is these differences in attenuation that allow us to see anatomic detail using X-rays.

5b. False
Hardening of the beam occurs when the beam is composed of a spectrum of wavelengths. The process of hardening occurs when lower energy photons are absorbed first, leaving more penetrating photons that will travel further through tissue.

5c. False
Digital radiography uses tubes of the same type of design as conventional radiography, where a spectrum or X-ray energies are produced with the maximum energy being set by the peak kilovoltage of an X-ray tube (kVp).

5d. True
Linear attenuation coefficient (μ) = 0.693/HVL.

5e. False
The reduction in the number of photons is exponential, and therefore never truly reaches zero. The intensity of the emerging beam can be calculated by $I = I_0 e^{-\mu d}$ where I is intensity, I_0 is initial intensity, μ is the attenuation coefficient and d is the thickness of material.

6a. False ****

X-ray beams used clinically are not monoenergetic. After one HVL the lower energy photons will have been preferentially removed and the beam will now be more penetrating. The second HVL of this beam will therefore be greater.

6b. True

The mass attenuation coefficient is obtained by dividing the linear attenuation coefficient by density; this makes it independent of density and relates only to atomic number and photon energy.

6c. False

Also known as coherent or Rayleigh scatter, this process refers to an interaction where a photon is deflected from a bound electron which is not ejected from the atom and therefore no ionizing events occur. For diagnostic energies, the probability of this effect is small compared to that of the Compton and photoelectric effects.

6d. True

The energy taken up by the photoelectron is absorbed very close (within ~ 1 μm) of the site of interaction.

6e. True

The photoelectric effect is proportional to Z^3/E^3 and is therefore more likely when low energy clinical beams interact with relatively high density contrast media.

7a. False ***

Intensity equals total photon energy in cross section per unit time. Removal of the characteristic rays would mean fewer photons.

7b. True

According to the inverse square law; if you double your distance, the area of the beam increases by four times, i.e. the intensity is reduced by 4. In the example given the distance is doubled twice, so intensity is reduced to one-sixteenth. Intensity is defined as energy transmitted per unit area.

7c. True

There is some attenuation in air but this is very low compared with the effect of the inverse square law.

7d. True

The operating kV is equal to the maximum photon energy possible; most photons will not be as energetic.

7e. False

Clinical X-ray beams are not monoenergetic; lower energy photons are more readily attenuated, so the beam intensity increases as it penetrates, thereby also increasing the HVL.

8a. True **

The Compton effect describes scatter, with a resulting recoil electron and scattered lower energy photon.

8b. False

This describes the photoelectric effect.

8c. True

Although the term 'free electrons' is used, it refers to any electron with a binding energy much lower than that of the incident photon.

8d. False
The Compton effect is proportional to the density of electrons, which is approximately proportional to the density of the tissue. The photoelectric effect is proportional to Z^3/E^3.

8e. False
The mass attenuation coefficient is already divided by the density of the tissue meaning the effect of density has been cancelled out. Also, the Compton effect is not proportional to atomic number. The linear attenuation coefficient of bone would be higher than that of soft tissue as the physical density, and thus the electron density is higher.

9a. False ***
The photoelectric effect cannot occur unless the photon has more energy than the binding energy of the electron. The photoelectric effect is at its maximum when the photon energy is just greater than the K-edge.

9b. True
The ejection of the photoelectron leaves a gap in the inner shell. An electron falling from an outer shell may give up some energy as characteristic radiation as it moves to a lower energy state.

9c. False
The high energy nature of this process causes that atom to become ionized, and the photoelectron continues on and collides to cause many more ionizations. As so many more ionization events are caused indirectly by the subsequent photoelectrons and Compton electrons, the direct biological damage from photon interactions is relatively small.

9d. False
The photoelectric effect is proportional to Z^3/E^3, and thus decreases with increasing photon energies.

9e. False
The energy of the incident photon is used to break the binding energy of the electron; its remaining energy is transferred to the photoelectron.

10a. False ***
The chance of the photoelectric effect is related to Z^3/E^3. In the human body at diagnostic X-ray levels the photoelectric effect occurs mainly at lower photon keV or with high atomic number contrast agents such as barium.

10b. False
In soft tissue interacting with a 30 keV beam approximately half the interactions will be Compton effect and half will be photoelectric. At lower keV the photoelectric effect predominates. At higher keV the Compton effect predominates.

10c. False
Pair production does not occur with photon energies of less than 1 MeV, and thus does not occur in diagnostic radiology.

10d. True
The electron can be scattered only forward or at angles of up to 90°.

10e. True

At very high photon energies the Compton effect begins to diminish, but at diagnostic radiology photon energies the Compton effect can be viewed as only dependent on the electron density, which is related to the density of the tissue.

11a. False ***

The outermost (lowest energy) layer is known as the valence band. The conduction band is the adjacent, higher energy band. On excitation of a phosphor, electrons in the valence band are energized and promoted to the conduction band.

11b. False

Between the valence band and conduction band is the forbidden zone. Impurities in the phosphor (deliberately manufactured in this way) contain electron bands which lie within the forbidden zone. Excited electrons which fall into these 'electron traps' subsequently move to the valence band with the release of light energy. This is the basis of photoluminescence.

11c. True

The energy absorbed is also proportional to the intensity of the beam itself.

11d. False

Computed radiography uses photostimulable phosphor plates. The detector plate is stimulated by light, usually a laser, to allow image formation.

11e. True

Optical stimulated luminescent dosimeters give readings down to 0.01 mSv. Unlike thermoluminescent dosimetry (TLDs), they can also be read more than once because not all electrons are released at the first reading by the scanning laser beam.

12a. True **

Most of the lower energy photons are absorbed either within the target, the tube wall or in the filter.

12b. False

K_α emission is emission of characteristic radiation after an electron falls from the L-shell to the K-shell. K_β emission occurs after an electron falls from the M-shell to the K-shell. Do not confuse K_α with an alpha particle.

12c. True

The energy of the photon and thus the wavelength and frequency ($E = hf$) is related to the energy difference of the electron between the shell it moves from and to.

12d. False

L-shell characteristic radiation is low energy radiation ($\sim$10 keV in the case of tungsten) that is unlikely to penetrate through the filter.

12e. False

Beta particles travel only very short distances and thus cannot be used for imaging. Beta particle emitters are sometimes used for therapy, e.g. thyroid ablation.

2. Radiation Hazards and Protection: Questions

1. Concerning biological effects of ionizing radiation:
   a. Most damage to cells occurs directly as a result of radiation striking and ionizing intracellular contents
   b. Linear energy transfer (LET) is defined as the energy deposited in tissue per unit path length
   c. Radiation with a high LET is more damaging to biological tissues
   d. Alpha particles have a much lower LET than beta particles
   e. Relative biological effectiveness (RBE) is the ratio of absorbed doses required to produce the same endpoint for two different radiation types

2. Regarding the interaction of ionizing radiation with tissue:
   a. Beta particles travel a few centimetres through human tissue before being fully absorbed
   b. The presence of water within living tissues is protective against the biological effects of radiation
   c. Ionizing radiation can directly damage the covalent bond of a deoxyribonucleic acid (DNA) molecule
   d. Proteins are relatively spared the effects of ionizing radiation
   e. The interaction of ionizing radiation with living tissue should only be used in medical practice in carrying out justified diagnostic procedures

3. Regarding radiation doses:
   a. Absorbed dose and kerma are the same
   b. The equivalent dose and absorbed dose are numerically identical for X-rays
   c. At low doses alpha particles have the same radiation effect for only 5% of the absorbed dose of X-rays
   d. The average background population dose in the UK is around 5 mSv/year
   e. Effective dose is primarily concerned with stochastic risk

4. Concerning effective dose:
   a. The effective dose of a barium enema is approximately twice that of a barium meal
   b. The tissue weighting factor is expressed in mGy/kg
   c. A posteroanterior (PA) chest radiograph has approximately the same effective dose as a 5-hour transatlantic flight
   d. Stomach and breast have the same tissue weighting factor
   e. It takes into account the differences in the risk of stochastic effects in different organs and tissues

9

5. **Absorbed dose, equivalent dose and effective dose:**
   a. Absorbed dose is measured in Gy, which is Jkg^{-1}
   b. Effective dose is the absorbed dose multiplied by a radiation weighting factor defined for each type of ionizing radiation
   c. Equivalent dose is the sum of the effective dose to each organ multiplied by a tissue weighting factor for each organ
   d. The radiation weighting factor for diagnostic X-ray radiation is 1
   e. The tissue weighting factor for colon is higher than that for thyroid

6. **Justification and optimization:**
   a. Only radiologists and radiographers are allowed to take the role of practitioner under Ionising Radiation (Medical Exposure) Regulations (IR(ME)R)
   b. It is possible for one person to be the referrer, practitioner and operator for an examination
   c. Optimization is the process of obtaining the best quality image possible
   d. The referrer is not responsible for justifying the radiation dose to the patient
   e. The practitioner has overall responsibility for compliance with IR(ME)R

7. **Annual dose limits:**
   a. The annual effective dose limit to the lens of the eye for an adult employee is 150 mSv
   b. The fetus of a pregnant employee should not receive more than 1 mSv over the declared term of pregnancy
   c. The annual effective dose limit for a member of the public is 1 mSv
   d. If a trainee is expected to receive more than a dose of 150 mSv to the hands they would have to be classified
   e. An employee receiving a radiological examination for medical purposes should inform their employer of the dose received so that it may be included in their annual dose limit

8. **Regarding risk from radiation:**
   a. Deterministic effects can occur at any dose
   b. Stochastic effects become more severe with increased dose
   c. The risk of fatal cancer in adults is 1 in 33 000 per mSv
   d. Cataracts are highly likely with an absorbed dose of 1 Gy to the eye
   e. Screening mammography carries a risk of 1 in 50 000 for fatal cancer

9. **Concerning deterministic effects of radiation:**
   a. The effect will only occasionally occur below the threshold dose
   b. The whole body fatal dose threshold is estimated to be 1 Gy
   c. Threshold dose for harming a developing fetus is approximately 0.1–0.5 mGy
   d. The severity of deterministic effects is not related to the dose
   e. Development of leukaemia in childhood has a threshold level of approximately 4 Sv to the bone marrow

10. **Concerning stochastic effects:**
    a. The risk of a stochastic effect increases exponentially with dose
    b. The risk of inducing a fatal cancer when exposing an adult patient to an effective dose of 10 mSv is 1 in 20 000
    c. Radiation induced fetal abnormality is an example of a stochastic effect
    d. By definition, stochastic effects must occur within one year
    e. Stochastic events arise by chance

11. **Concerning carcinogenesis as a result of radiation:**
    a. Radiation induced carcinogenesis is a stochastic effect
    b. The risk of inducing a fatal cancer for a computed tomography (CT) of the abdomen is approximately 1 in 2000
    c. A CT head has a lower stochastic risk than a CT of the abdomen partly because brain tissue has a lower risk factor of developing cancer than many organs in the abdomen
    d. Carcinogenesis follows a latent period, with a peak of approximately 7 years for leukaemia and 40 years or more for solid tumours
    e. The risk of developing a fatal cancer following radiation exposure is not related to patient age

12. **Medical radiation doses:**
    a. The typical effective dose for a radionuclide bone scan is 5 mSv
    b. The typical effective dose for a CT head is 2 mSv
    c. The typical effective dose for a PA chest X-ray (CXR) is 0.5 mSv
    d. The effective dose for most examinations is higher for antero-posterior (AP) than for PA radiographs
    e. The effective dose should never be higher than the diagnostic reference level for the examination

13. **The average population dose of radiation:**
    a. Endogenous radioactive substances within the body contribute a negligible amount to our total annual radiation dose
    b. Natural background radiation is mainly as a result of cosmic radiation
    c. Medical exposures account for approximately 15% of annual radiation to the UK population
    d. Nuclear fallout from weapons testing is a significant source of background radiation in the UK
    e. On average an individual in Cornwall will be subjected to less background radiation than an individual in other parts of the UK

14. Radiation protection legislation:
a. Ionising Radiations Regulations 1999 (IRR99) apply to patients, staff and the general public
b. Breaches of IR(ME)R can be dealt with under criminal law
c. The Health Protection Agency enforces IRR99
d. Medicines (Administration of Radioactive Substances) Regulations 1978 (MARS) state that for an individual to administer a radionuclide to a patient they must have been granted an Administration of Radioactive Substances Advisory Committee (ARSAC) licence
e. The employee has overall responsibility for compliance under IR(ME)R

15. Under the IRR99:
a. The employer has to consult a radiation protection supervisor (RPS) to ensure compliance with the regulations
b. An area must be deemed controlled if an employee were likely to receive more than 150 mSv to their hands over the course of a working year
c. New X-ray equipment only requires testing after the manufacturer's warranty has expired
d. There is no requirement for patient dose assessment; these are the remit of IR(ME)R
e. There is no obligation to report an incident where a patient receives double the intended dose in a CT examination if it occurs due to human error

16. Concerning IRR99:
a. An employer must notify the Health and Safety Executive (HSE) of its intention to install all new pieces of radiological equipment
b. The radiation protection advisor (RPA) and the RPS is often the same person
c. It is the manufacturer's responsibility to perform a prior risk assessment before installing a new piece of radiological equipment
d. The annual dose limit for the lens of the eye is 150 mSv
e. A female member of staff must not receive an annual dose of more than 13 mSv

17. The IRR99:
a. Aims to minimize harmful ionizing radiation to patients
b. Breaches of the Approved Code of Practice (ACOP) will lead to prosecution
c. A dose constraint is three-tenths of an employee's dose limit
d. An RPA is responsible for optimization of radiological examinations
e. An RPS is normally a medical physicist

18. **More IRR99:**
    a. IRR99 makes allowance for paediatric nurses who exceed their dose limit when accompanying a young child for a radionuclide study as long as they are a designated comforter or carer
    b. Written rules relating to people who work in controlled or supervised areas are issued to individual departments by representatives of the Health and Safety Commission
    c. Local rules are only necessary for controlled areas
    d. These regulations describe the need for a contingency plan should there be a 'reasonably foreseeable' chance of an uncontrolled exposure to radiation
    e. Radiation protection is the sole responsibility of the RPA

19. **Regarding radiological examinations:**
    a. The maximum activity of radiopharmaceuticals that can be administered is kept within limits that are set at local level by the ARSAC certificate holder at an institution
    b. The practitioner must have passed the Fellow of the Royal College of Radiologists (FRCR) part 1 examination
    c. IR(ME)R state that the operator has overall responsibility for compliance with the regulations
    d. An operator must be a health-care professional
    e. Justification for the examination is given by the referrer

20. **IR(ME)R 2000:**
    a. IR(ME)R apply to patients undergoing medical treatment, health screening and occupational health surveys, but not to medico-legal procedures or research programmes
    b. If a patient receives 10 times the intended dose for a CXR the incident needs to be reported to the HSE
    c. Ionizing radiation doses must be kept as low as is reasonably practicable (ALARP)
    d. There is no dose constraint for individuals being examined for research purposes under IR(ME)R
    e. A trainee is not legally allowed to participate in practical aspects of an examination

21. **Concerning diagnostic reference levels (DRLs):**
    a. DRLs for selected radiological examinations are set nationally
    b. If a patient receives a dose greater than the DRL, the employer must report this to the IR(ME)R inspectorate
    c. DRL in radionuclide imaging is expressed in activity administered
    d. The employer must audit local DRLs
    e. Aging equipment is a justified reason to exceed DRLs

22. Radiological examination of female patients:

a. For most radiographic examinations the 28-day rule is sufficient

b. The 28-day rule involves asking the patient if she could be pregnant and proceeding if she states she could not be, and if her last period was less than 28 days ago

c. The 10-day rule involves scheduling the examination no more than 10 days after the patient's last menstrual period (LMP)

d. A CT scan of the pelvis may cause fetal damage such as limb abnormalities

e. The use of ionizing radiation in women known to be pregnant is illegal under IR(ME)R

23. Controlled and supervised areas:

a. A controlled area is required if any individual other than the patient is likely to receive an effective dose greater than 6 mSv or more than three-tenths of any equivalent dose limit

b. A controlled area must have special working procedures in order to restrict exposure

c. Controlled areas must be shielded with at least 2 mm of lead lining

d. A supervised area is required if the dose levels are not sufficient to require designation as a controlled area but it is possible an individual could receive an effective dose greater than 1 mSv

e. Controlled areas should be clearly marked with warning signs describing the radiation source and hazard (for example, external source or contamination)

24. Other legislation:

a. The Medical and Dental Guidance Notes are guidelines that are compliant with the overall requirement set out in IRR99

b. The International Commission on Radiological Protection (ICRP) is ultimately responsible for governing the use of radiation in medical practice

c. The Health and Safety at Work Act 1974 (HSWA) and the Medicines Act are the two areas of UK legislation that cover all medical radiation use

d. Individual dose limits for diagnostic radionuclide imaging procedures are set out by the Radioactive Substances Act 1993 (RSA)

e. The RSA states that all radioactive waste emitted from a patient undergoing a medical procedure must be packaged and sealed in an appropriately labelled disposal receptacle

25. **Radiation equipment standards:**
   a. Total filtration of the beam should be at least 2.5 mm equivalent of aluminium for most exposures
   b. All exposure switches should require positive pressure to maintain continuous exposure
   c. The required warning signal when an X-ray beam is switched on is an audible warning
   d. Leakage from the X-ray tube should not be greater than 1 Gy in one hour at one metre from the focus
   e. Actual kV of the beam should be ± 5 kV of the kV selected on the control panel

26. **Regarding personal protective equipment:**
   a. The employer is responsible for providing personal protective equipment such as lead aprons, thyroid shields, leaded glasses and screens
   b. Lead aprons of 3.5 mm lead are commonly used in fluoroscopy and intervention
   c. Lead aprons provide an acceptable protection from the primary beam
   d. Lead screens should be positioned between the operator and the X-ray tube in fluoroscopy and intervention
   e. In most circumstances a dosimeter should be worn under a lead apron

27. **Measuring dose:**
   a. Measurements of air kerma may be undertaken to represent absorbed dose in tissue
   b. Ionization chambers are more sensitive when they are smaller
   c. Dose area product (DAP) is measured as dose in gray per unit area
   d. Thermoluminescent dosimetry (TLD) may be used to monitor patient dose
   e. Optically stimulated luminescence (OSL) personal dosimeters use filters to prolong their useful life

28. **Dosimeters:**
   a. Film dosimeters are cheap and provide a permanent record of exposure
   b. TLDs are more expensive than film, but are far more sensitive
   c. TLDs have minimal energy dependence for diagnostic X-rays and are less susceptible to environmental effects such as heat and humidity than film
   d. Deep and shallow doses can be estimated with both film and TLD personal dosimetry
   e. Electronic dosimeters are very sensitive and provide immediate readings

2. Radiation Hazards and Protection: Answers

1a. False **

Most damage occurs indirectly as a result of ionization of water molecules (the human body being 75% water), with the ions going on to damage other molecules such as DNA and proteins.

1b. True

LET gives a measure of how concentrated the energy deposition is for different types of ionizing radiation, with high LET energy types causing multiple ionizations close together and thus more likely to damage both strands of DNA molecules.

1c. True

A high LET radiation will deposit all of its energy in a smaller area of tissue than a radiation with a low LET. This concentration of energy is more likely to cause damage.

1d. False

Alpha particles have a much greater mass than beta particles and for the same initial energy travel a much smaller distance; they impart their energy over distances such as a single strand of DNA, resulting in a much greater chance of irreparable biological genetic damage.

1e. True

The radiation weighting factors that are used to calculate equivalent dose are based on the RBE at low doses for other types of radiation compared with X-rays.

2a. False **

Beta particles are electrons that travel only a few millimetres before being absorbed.

2b. False

The presence of water accounts for indirect cellular damage in the presence of ionizing radiation. When irradiated, it produces a hydroxyl free radical which is a powerful oxidizing agent.

2c. True

This is one of the biological effects of ionizing radiation.

2d. False

Proteins are particularly susceptible to direct damage from ionizing radiation (e.g. covalent bond, enzymes).

2e. False

Therapeutic agents such as radiopharmaceuticals or radiotherapy exploit the interaction of ionizing radiation with living tissue to good effect.

3a. False *

In diagnostic radiology they can be used interchangeably, but at high energies there is more spread within the material, i.e. the energy deposited per unit mass (absorbed dose) will then differ from that released to matter (kerma).

3b. True

The sievert and gray are the special names for equivalent and absorbed doses and are both used instead of Jkg^{-1}.

3c. True

The weighting factor for calculating the equivalent dose of alpha particles is 20.

3d. False

More like 2.2 mSv in a year; this varies depending on the area of the country and the local prevalence of igneous rock. The average background radiation in Cornwall is more than twice the national average at approximately 7 mSv per year.

3e. True

Weighting factors take account of differing tissue sensitivities.

4a. True **

A barium meal is 1.5−3 mSv, a barium enema is 3−6 mSv.

4b. False

It is a factor so has no units. Organs are divided into low, medium and high risk and the total adds up to 1.0.

4c. True

Effective dose of a PA chest radiograph is approximately 0.01−0.025 mSv. Air flight has an effective dose of approximately 0.004 mSv per hour.

4d. True

They are both high risk.

4e. True

This is achieved by incorporating the tissue weighting factor for all irradiated organs.

5a. True *

The gray is the special name given to the unit of absorbed dose and is equal to Jkg^{-1}. Likewise the sievert, the unit for equivalent and effective dose, has the same dimensions but has been given a separate special name in the SI system to distinguish it from absorbed dose.

5b. False

This describes equivalent dose.

5c. False

This describes effective dose.

5d. True

For diagnostic X-rays, gray and sievert can almost be used interchangeably. The weighting factor for particles may be much greater than for X-rays; e.g. for alpha particles it is 20.

5e. True

The tissue weighting factors were revised in 2006. These revised values are: Gonads 0.08 (previously 0.2), Red bone marrow 0.12, Colon 0.12, Lung 0.12, Stomach 0.12, Bladder 0.04 (previously 0.05), Breast 0.12 (previously 0.05), Liver 0.04 (previously 0.05), Oesophagus 0.04 (previously 0.05), Thyroid 0.04 (previously 0.05), Skin 0.01, Bone surfaces 0.01, Brain 0.01 (previously without a separate listing), Salivary glands 0.01 (previously without a separate listing), and Remainder 0.12 (previously 0.05).

6a. False **
The role of practitioner can be performed by any health-care professional who has had adequate training and is entitled by the employer to be able to carry out this duty. Practitioners may include radiologists, radiographers, cardiologists and dentists.

6b. True
Commonly dentists would perform all three roles.

6c. False
Optimization is the process of producing an image that is suitable for the clinical purpose at a dose ALARP.

6d. True
The duties of the referrer are to provide the patient's name and identification details, the LMP if necessary, and enough clinical details for the practitioner to justify the examination. The employer should provide the referrer with referral criteria that indicate the clinical circumstances in which particular examinations may be justified.

6e. False
The employer has overall responsibility for compliance.

7a. False **
Doses to parts of the body are listed as equivalent doses. Effective dose limits refer to the stochastic chance of developing cancer and are for the whole body.

7b. True
This limit applies to the declared term: from when the employee informs her employer that she is pregnant until delivery of her child.

7c. True
This is equivalent to less than half the UK background dose.

7d. False
Trainees cannot be classified. Employees need to be classified if the effective dose is likely to exceed 6 mSv or three-tenths of any equivalent dose. In order to be classified an employee has to be over the age of 18 and be certified as medically fit to be classified.

7e. False
Annual dose limits only refer to the radiation received as part of employment. They do not include background radiation or radiation justified on medical grounds.

8a. False ***
Deterministic effects will only occur if a threshold is reached.

8b. False
Stochastic effects either happen or they do not. Beyond threshold dose deterministic effects become more severe with increased dose.

8c. False
This is the risk of childhood cancer following irradiation in utero. In adults it is 1 in 20 000 per mSv.

8d. False
The threshold for this deterministic effect is between 2 and 6 Gy. It is cumulative over a person's lifetime.

8e. True
Clinical use of ionizing radiation is never without risk.

9a. False **

The effect will not occur below the threshold dose.

9b. False

The whole body fatal dose threshold is approximately 2–5 Gy.

9c. False

The threshold for fetal harm in utero is 0.1–0.5 Gy.

9d. False

The severity of deterministic effects is related to the dose.

9e. False

Development of cancer as a result of radiation is a stochastic effect.

10a. False ***

The risk increases linearly. This is known as the linear no threshold theory.

10b. False

The risk is 5% per Sv, or 1 in 20 000 per mSv. An effective dose of 10 mSv therefore carries a risk of 1 in 2000.

10c. False

It is a deterministic effect.

10d. False

There is a latency period between the radiation exposure and the effect; generally at least 5 years and for cancers it may be in excess of 40 years. Genetic effects may only be seen in future generations.

10e. True

Stochastic means statistical in nature.

11a. True **

This means the likelihood of development is governed by chance.

11b. True

The risk is 5% per Sv for an adult between about 20 and 60 years old. A 10 mSv CT scan would therefore carry a risk of 1 in 2000. Note that this is the risk of developing a fatal cancer. The chance of developing cancer is higher than this.

11c. True

The weighting factor for brain tissue is 0.01. Stomach and colon by comparison all have values of 0.12.

11d. True

The consequence of this is that the risk of fatal cancer is much lower for the elderly population who are the most commonly scanned in the hospital setting, as they are likely to reach the end of their natural lives before the development of a solid tumour.

11e. False

For a child the risk is approximately three times greater than for a 40-year-old.

12a. True ***

Some radionuclide scans can incur large effective doses, particularly those that accumulate throughout the body, e.g. labelled white blood cell for occult infection.

12b. True

A CT head is approximately 2 mSv, a CT abdomen/pelvis 10–20 mSv, and a CT thorax 8 mSv.

12c. False

A CXR has an effective dose of approximately 0.015 mSv.

12d. True

This occurs as many organs that are more sensitive to radiation lie anteriorly in the body and thus receive unattenuated beam and consequently a higher dose in AP radiographs.

12e. False

Diagnostic reference levels are for audit purposes and are given for a standard patient. Some particularly larger individuals may require 10 or more times the normal dose of radiation for the detector plate or film to receive enough radiation to produce an adequate image.

13a. False **

Potassium-40 is an isotope with a very long half-life. It contributes to 60% of our internal radiation. Internal sources account for approximately 12% of our annual background radiation.

13b. False

Half the annual background radiation is from radon and it is variations in radon exposure that give rise to very high background doses in different geographical regions. Cosmic radiation accounts for 10%.

13c. True

Although there are obviously very big population variations in medical exposure since most people receive no more than a dental X-ray in a typical year.

13d. False

It accounts for less than 1%.

13e. False

Cornwall has the highest background radiation due to radon in the rock. The average annual dose is 7 mSv (UK average is 2.2 mSv).

14a. False **

IRR99 only apply to staff and the public at large. Patients are protected under IR(ME)R.

14b. True

Radiation protection is rightly taken seriously.

14c. False

IRR99 are enforced by the HSE.

14d. False

The ARSAC licence covers an individual doctor but administration of radionuclides to patients can be performed by suitably trained individuals on behalf of the ARSAC licence holder.

14e. False

This is the position of the employer.

15a. False ***
An RPA must be consulted on compliance.

15b. True
An area must be controlled if an employee is likely to receive more than three-tenths of any dose limit, if there are procedures in place to limit exposure, or if an average daily dose may exceed 7.5 μSvh^{-1}.

15c. False
A critical examination of any new equipment needs to be carried out prior to its first use; this is the responsibility of the installer, while other commissioning tests should be carried out by the employer as the basis of the ongoing quality assurance (QA) programme.

15d. False
IRR99 also require patient dose assessment.

15e. True
Doubling of an intended CT dose is not necessarily notifiable under IR(ME)R if this occurs due to a failure to follow written procedures. If it were due to an equipment fault, it would be reportable under IRR99.

16a. False **
The employer must state their intention to use ionizing radiation on a site for the first time; thereafter no further notification is needed unless there is a change in the type of work being carried out.

16b. False
The RPA is usually a medical physicist. The RPS, in radiology, is usually a senior radiographer.

16c. False
It is the employer's responsibility to perform a prior risk assessment.

16d. True
This is because the threshold dose for cataract is approximately 5 Sv. If an employee works for 35 years they should not exceed this level.

16e. False
A female employee should not receive an abdominal dose of more than 13 mSv in a consecutive 3-month period. This should never be an issue in medical practice.

17a. False **
IRR99 relate to the safety of employees at work. IR(ME)R relate to patients.

17b. False
ACOP is published by the Health and Safety Commission, the same body that regulates IRR99. ACOP provides practical guidance for complying with the law under IRR99. Although ACOP is not legally binding in itself, it provides guidance on how compliance with the regulations may be achieved.

17c. False
Dose constraints are local limits placed on exposures to patients, staff who do not use radiation, or, under special circumstances, carers. They are not dose limits which are legally enforceable and refer to workers or the general public, but not to patients.

17d. False

An RPA is normally a medical physicist who is consulted by the employer and advises on compliance with IRR99 including designation of controlled areas, local rules, planning of installations and acceptance of equipment and instigating QA programmes.

17e. False

In radiology departments, an RPS is normally a senior radiographer and is responsible under the employer for supervising adherence to local rules, including risk assessments, arranging for staff doses to be monitored, investigations of excessive dose and monitoring and performing QA programmes.

18a. False ***

IRR99 permit the dose limit of the public to be relaxed for comforters and carers so that they can accompany certain patients into situations where they will be exposed to radiation. In practice this is almost always the parents of children who are undergoing radionuclide examinations. The employer can choose to override the dose limit for a member of the public (1 mSv) but must set a dose constraint (usually up to 5 mSv) and must explain the risk to the parents. Employees cannot be classified as comforters or carers in this context.

18b. False

Rules and work procedures of individual departments are set locally, usually with the advice of the employer's RPA. They will be based on the requirements of the IRR99 and the Health and Safety Commission ACOP.

18c. False

Local rules may also be required for supervised areas.

18d. True

The chance of such an occurrence should be assessed in the prior risk assessment. For X-ray use the contingency plan may be no more than arrangements to ensure that equipment is switched off and not used again until it has been repaired by an engineer.

18e. False

The RPA's responsibility is only to advise. Responsibility for radiation protection rests with the employer.

19a. False ***

These limits are set nationally. In the UK they are set by ARSAC on behalf of the Department of Health.

19b. False

The practitioner requires theoretical knowledge of radiation protection and imaging techniques but may include cardiologists, dentists and radiographers.

19c. False

The employer has overall responsibility and should have written procedures in place.

19d. False

The term 'operator' includes a wide range of people performing the different roles involved in obtaining the medical exposure. They must be suitably trained to carry out their particular role.

19e. False

Adequate clinical information must be given by the referrer but justification is given by the practitioner.

20a. False **

IR(ME)R apply to all examinations for medical purposes, including medical diagnosis and treatment, health screening, health surveys, medico-legal examinations, and research.

20b. False

For low dose examinations the exposure would have to be 20 times the intended amount to be legally reportable. A local investigation should be undertaken anyway.

20c. True

Note the word practicable is used instead of possible or achievable. Financial, time and other constraints may mean that even though it would be possible to give a lower dose, a higher dose may be given if it would not be reasonably practicable to perform the study in a way to give the lower dose.

20d. False

Dose constraints are set through ethics committees for each research project and should be strictly adhered to.

20e. False

A trainee may participate in practical aspects of the examination if supervised by someone who has the adequate training.

21a. True ***

The employer must set local DRLs through patient dose audit. The local value should not be greater than the national value.

21b. False

They are not used to determine whether a dose to a particular patient is too high since there is a large variation in dose between patients due to size, etc.

21c. True

ARSAC provide guidance for national DRLs.

21d. True

This is a requirement under IR(ME)R. It is also a requirement to investigate incidents in which the DRL is consistently exceeded.

21e. False

This is not a valid excuse for exceeding national DRLs.

22a. True ***

The 10-day rule is now considered unnecessarily restrictive as the risk of pregnancy for most women who state they are not pregnant and whose LMP is less than 28 days ago is small.

22b. True

This is the preferred method of excluding pregnancy prior to most radiological procedures.

22c. True

The 10-day rule is not often used now, but might be considered for example for a high dose examination such as CT on a woman who is currently trying to get pregnant. Consideration should also be given to whether or not the scan will be done anyway if the patient is subsequently found to be pregnant at the time of her next due period. If the scan cannot be safely delayed 9 months, it would be safer to perform the scan as early as possible during the pregnancy.

22d. False

A single CT abdomen would give a dose in the order of 10–20 mGy to the fetus. The deterministic threshold for fetal abnormalities is not less than 100 mGy and is possibly higher.

22e. False

Even if the patient is known to be pregnant a scan can be justified if the clinical risks of not performing the scan are greater.

23a. True ***

Note the use of the words 'likely to receive'. A controlled area is also designated if the dose rate could exceed 7.5 μSvh^{-1} averaged over the working day.

23b. True

This is generally contained within the Local Rules.

23c. False

There is no legal requirement on shielding. For mobile sets a distance of 2 m is normally sufficient via the inverse square law to reduce the radiation to levels not requiring a controlled area. Barium plasterboard, or even normal bricks and mortar all reduce the energy of the radiation and can be all that is required. For higher radiation energies, such as positron emitters used for positron emission tomography (PET), the shielding required is likely to be greater than 2 mm lead.

23d. True

Such an area should have its exposure conditions under review in case of change.

23e. True

Information should include the type of radiation and how a person entering the area could be affected.

24a. True ****

In addition to guidance on compliance with IRR99 the Medical and Dental Guidance Notes include advice on compliance with IR(ME)R and RSA.

24b. False

The ICRP have published recommendations that formed the basis of European directives and UK legislation relating to radiation protection; in particular the justification and optimization of radiological exposures and the concept of dose limits. They have no judicial role in their implementation.

24c. True

The Health and Safety at Work Act 1974 (HSWA) covers all radiation use in a legal context and the two groups that work under its rules.

The Health and Safety Commission is responsible for producing guidelines covering employers, employees and the public. The HSE polices the legislation; ICRP recommendations, European directives, IR(ME)R and IRR99 form the basis of this legislation. MARS however are not part of HSWA; they are enacted under the Medicines Act.

24d. False

Maximum activities that may be administered in normal circumstances are determined by ARSAC. The RSA is concerned with the protection of the general population and the environment and governs the disposal of radioactive substances by hospitals. It is regulated by the Environment Agency in England and Wales and by the equivalent devolved agencies in Scotland and Northern Ireland.

24e. False

Limitations are placed on the total amount of radioactive waste but individual types need only be managed appropriately to minimize risk to the public, staff and environment. For example, gaseous waste from lung studies should be exhausted to an area exterior of the building. In general there is no restriction on excreted waste because the dilution factor in the sewerage system is sufficient to cause minimal environmental impact. In hospitals, however, designated toilets should be used to minimize the risk of the spread of contamination.

25a. True **

An exception to this is in dental radiography of less than 70 keV where the requirement is 1.5 mm of aluminium.

25b. False

This is true for fluoroscopy and radiography but exception is made for CT scanning when the scan sequence can be initiated with a single button press.

25c. False

A visible warning light to indicate that the X-ray beam is switched on is a requirement although an additional audible warning is common, particularly for radiographic sets.

25d. False

This would be grossly high. Leakage should not be greater than 1 mGy in 1 hour at 1 metre.

25e. True

This can be checked by assessing the beam dose directly.

26a. True ***

The operator is obliged to use the equipment that is specified in the Local Rules for controlled areas.

26b. False

0.35 mm of lead or lead equivalent is common. Many modern aprons use barium and other lower atomic number materials in place of lead as the K-edge absorption produces more attenuation of the beam for a lighter apron for most energies of X-rays used in diagnostic radiology.

26c. False

Lead aprons provide protection from scatter, but they are not adequate protection against the primary beam.

26d. False

If the beam is correctly collimated and the operator is not standing within the path of the primary or transmitted beam, then the vast majority of the radiation reaching the operator is scatter from the patient. Therefore the screen should be placed between the operator and the patient, not between the operator and tube.

26e. True

This allows the dosimeter to record a reading of effective dose delivered to the body of the operator. In some circumstances dosimeters should be worn outside personal protective equipment; ring dosimeters for monitoring equivalent dose to the operator's fingers would be an example.

27a. False ***

Generally dosimeters are calibrated in terms of air kerma. Although the atomic numbers of air and soft tissue are very similar, conversion factors are needed to convert the measurements to absorbed dose to water, but these are not generally applied to diagnostic radiology.

27b. False

Sensitivity is proportional to volume.

27c. False

DAP is the *product* of dose in gray and area, e.g. $Gycm^2$.

27d. True

TLDs can be used to measure entrance surface dose in radiography.

27e. False

The doses behind the different filters are used to estimate deep and shallow personal dose equivalent.

28a. True **

Film dosimeters, however, have significant disadvantages such as a response which is highly dependent on radiation energy and are affected by environmental conditions such as heat and humidity.

28b. False

The sensitivity of film and TLDs is approximately equal, having minimum readings of between 0.1 and 0.2 mSv.

28c. True

These are the main advantages of TLDs over film. Because of the lack of susceptibility to environmental conditions they may be used for longer monitoring periods, e.g. 3 months.

28d. True

Filters are used to estimate different depths. For TLDs a different TLD chip is required under each filter if deep and shallow dose are to be measured.

28e. True

Electronic dosimeters are far more expensive, but are sensitive to approximately 1 µSv and give direct readings.

3. Imaging with X-rays: Questions

1. **Regarding the use of contrast media:**
   a. Radio-opaque contrast media agents are chosen because their atomic number is chosen to maximize the absorption of a diagnostic X-ray beam by the Compton effect
   b. The absorption energy/K-edge of iodine is 53 keV
   c. Bone and iodine demonstrate a similar computed tomography (CT) number because they have a similar atomic number
   d. High density and low density contrast agents can be administered together in certain circumstances to improve image contrast and quality
   e. A positive contrast agent should ideally have K-edge energy equal to the characteristic radiation emitted from the X-ray tube

2. **Concerning factors that affect radiation dose:**
   a. The entrance surface dose of an anteroposterior (AP) pelvic X-ray is approximately 10 times greater than the dose to the imaging plate
   b. To achieve a similar dose to the imaging plate, an 85 kV beam will result in a greater entrance surface dose than a 65 kV beam
   c. Additional beam filtration generally improves image quality but increases the patient dose
   d. Increasing the focus–detector distance reduces the dose to the patient
   e. The use of an anti-scatter grid can reduce the dose to the patient

3. **Contrast and spatial resolutions:**
   a. Spatial resolution may be measured in line pairs per millimetre
   b. Spatial resolution is unaffected by the contrast of the objects being imaged
   c. Image quality refers to spatial resolution but not to contrast resolution
   d. Contrast is the ability to differentiate between structures within the image
   e. Subject contrast increases with an increased thickness of the imaged organ

4. **Imaging geometry:**
   a. Distortion is greater with a larger focus–film distance
   b. Geometrical unsharpness occurs with round-edged objects
   c. Object–film distance is directly related to unsharpness
   d. Magnification in mammography is achieved by increasing object–film distance
   e. An ideal set-up would minimize focal spot size, maximize focus–film distance and minimize object–film distance

5. **Unsharpness:**
   a. Screen unsharpness is the product of movement unsharpness and geometric unsharpness
   b. Geometric unsharpness can be reduced by the use of an air gap
   c. Movement unsharpness is approximately equal to the speed of movement of the object multiplied by the time of exposure
   d. Absorption or edge unsharpness is produced around the edge of a tapered or rounded structure such as a blood vessel
   e. Movement unsharpness can be a significant problem in mammography due to longer exposure times

6. **Noise and signal to noise ratio (SNR):**
   a. Quantum noise or mottle is due to random variation in the number of photons being detected
   b. Electronic noise is predominant in CT
   c. Noise is commonly expressed as a proportion of the total number of photons detected in a single area or pixel (M), as $1/M^{1/2}$
   d. SNR is defined as $M/M^{1/2}$
   e. Structural noise is caused by random background radiation from the patient and structures near the film or detector plate

7. **The quality of the X-ray beam is hardened by:**
   a. Increasing the tube kV
   b. Decreasing the focus to film distance
   c. Increased thickness of aluminium filter
   d. Increasing the tube mA
   e. Increased thickness of the intensifying screen

8. **Scatter and grids:**
   a. Scatter predominantly affects spatial resolution
   b. Increasing the kV reduces the scatter reaching the plate or detector
   c. Grid techniques reduce scatter reaching the film or plate
   d. Grid techniques increase image contrast resolution
   e. Grid techniques reduce patient dose

9. **Use of compression:**
   a. Reduces attenuation of the beam
   b. Reduces scatter
   c. Reduces contrast seen in the organ being imaged
   d. Requires a high kV technique
   e. Is only used in mammography

10. Tubes and heating:
a. X-ray tubes contain a cathode and an anode
b. The electron beam is emitted from the anode after bombardment of the target
c. An increase in angle of the target decreases the effective focal spot size
d. The focusing cup refers to the target area of the anode
e. Heat loading of the tube is the product of kV and mAs and is measured in joules

11. For rotating anodes:
a. The rotator bearings are lubricated with a metal such as silver
b. The anode mainly loses heat via conduction through a molybdenum (Mo) stem
c. The anode completes one full rotation in the exposure time to evenly spread the heat along the focal spot track
d. The edge of the anode disk is rounded
e. Typical effective focal spot sizes would be 0.6–1 mm for general radiography and 0.1–0.4 mm for mammography

12. Concerning generators:
a. Three phase generators produce a higher kVp than single phase generators
b. Single phase generators require longer exposure times for the same kVp and mA settings
c. Modern high frequency generators produce a relatively stable voltage so kV can be assumed to be equal to kVp
d. Self rectifying generators are used in modern X-ray equipment and produce a higher mean kV than three phase generators
e. High frequency generators produce a harder more penetrating beam at the same kVp

13. In quality control of X-ray equipment and procedures:
a. At 70 kV a half-value layer (HVL) of 2.5 mm aluminium would be expected if there was adequate filtration
b. kV can be measured using a penetrameter
c. A Leeds test object is used for quality control in fluoroscopy
d. Quality assurance (QA) for lead aprons may include taking an X-ray image of them to check the lead lining is intact
e. The image distortion of an image intensifier can be assessed using a rectangular grid

14. **Further QA of X-ray equipment and procedures:**
    a. A densitometer measures the density of anode target material
    b. A QA programme should ensure that tests are done consistently at agreed time intervals according to a written protocol
    c. Audit is a requirement of QA
    d. Discrepancies of up to 10 mm of collimation of a 20 cm square test plate at 1 m would be acceptable
    e. Different dose area product (DAP) values for similar examinations may indicate a difference in the equipment or the operators

15. **Film chemistry:**
    a. Film emulsion is a suspension of silver halide crystals
    b. Film for general radiology normally consists of a polyester base with an emulsion backing on one side
    c. The film emulsion layer is only approximately 0.5 mm thick
    d. Each crystal is about 1 μm diameter
    e. The emulsion is only responsive to ionizing radiation of about 1 keV and above

16. **More film chemistry:**
    a. Gamma depends on the variation in crystal size
    b. Gamma increases with temperature and developer concentration
    c. A high gamma film has a wide latitude
    d. Development of the film involves reduction of the silver ions by an acid fixing agent
    e. A brown vinegary film may be caused by inadequate washing

17. **Speed, density and noise:**
    a. Speed is equal to 1000 divided by the air kerma (in μGy) required for density 1 above base plus fog
    b. Typical speed for a rare earth film–screen combination would be about 400
    c. Quantum sink refers to the random attenuation of X-ray photons in the patient causing scatter
    d. Optical density (OD) of film is $\log_{10}$ (transmitted light/incident light)
    e. An OD of 5–10 would be typical for bony structures on an adequately exposed film

18. **Film–screen:**
    a. Rare earth materials are used for intensifying screens as their K-edges are in the diagnostic range
    b. Intensifying screens utilize thermoluminescence
    c. Up to two intensifying screens might be used
    d. Characteristic curves are plotted with OD against exposure
    e. Film gamma is measured as the average slope of the characteristic curve

19. **Further film–screen:**
    a. An acceptable level of base plus fog has an OD of 0.5
    b. A film–screen combination with a high gamma will have a relatively wide latitude
    c. Ideally an intensification screen should be as thick as possible
    d. A phosphor with greater X-rays to light conversion will be associated with more noise than an equally sensitive phosphor with a lower conversion efficiency but a greater thickness
    e. Crossover is impossible if a single side of film emulsion is used

20. **Intensifying screens:**
    a. Intensifying screens reduce dose but increase noise for the same amount of film blackening
    b. Without an intensification screen, only about 20% of the X-ray photons would be absorbed by the film
    c. Intensification factor is the ratio of kerma for a film density of 1 with and without the intensifying screen
    d. Rare earth screens are used because of their very high atomic number
    e. A thicker phosphor layer decreases dose required at the expense of greater noise and screen unsharpness

21. **In mammography:**
    a. A K-edge filter such as molybdenum is commonly used
    b. The filter should not be the same element as the anode target otherwise the characteristic radiation would be absorbed
    c. Typical spatial resolution for both digital and film mammography is 15 lp/mm
    d. Typical mean glandular breast dose is 1.5–3 mGy for a single exposure
    e. Typical kV for mammography is 24–35 kV

22. **With linear tomography:**
    a. Blurring is deliberately introduced into the image through movement
    b. The cut plane slice is centred at the pivot height
    c. The slice thickness is increased by increasing the angle of movement of the tube and plate
    d. Zonography techniques image a very narrow slice thickness
    e. Contrast is typically lower in linear tomography compared to conventional radiography because of the blurring of overlying tissues spread over the image

23. **Concerning dual energy radiography:**
    a. Images are taken in rapid succession, alternating between a high tube current and a low tube current to allow the formation of a subtracted image that maximizes tissue contrast
    b. For a given mA, soft tissue contrast will be increased by using a lower kV X-ray beam
    c. Subtracting a low kV image from a high kV image will improve soft tissue contrast and minimize the visualization of bone
    d. The detection of a calcified lung nodule could be improved by subtracting the low kV image from the high kV image
    e. Dual energy digital subtraction angiography (otherwise known as DE DSA) is performed after an intra-arterial or intravenous injection of iodinated contrast medium

3. Imaging with X-rays: Answers

1a. False ***

Radio-opaque contrast media is chosen so that the high atomic number maximizes photoelectric absorption of the beam. The K-edge energy of the contrast medium should be slightly less than the major part of the X-ray energy spectrum to maximize this effect.

1b. False

The atomic number of iodine is 53; its K-edge energy is 33 keV.

1c. False

The atomic number of iodine is 53. The atomic number of bone is approximately 13. In tissues, CT number is related to electron density which itself is closely related to physical density. However, in higher Z materials such as iodine there is significant attenuation due to the photoelectric effect and therefore iodine will have a higher CT number than bone even though the physical density is less than that of bone.

1d. True

An example is a barium enema, where barium and air are used to demonstrate the mucosal anatomy of the colon. Air is used much less as a contrast agent in other areas of radiology since the introduction of CT and magnetic resonance imaging (MRI).

1e. False

The K-edge should be slightly less than the beam energy. If they are exactly the same then the contrast media will not attenuate the beam. Substances are relatively 'transparent' to X-rays with energy just below their K-edge. This property is utilized when filtering X-ray beams.

2a. False ***

The entrance surface dose of a pelvic X-ray is far greater than 10 times the exit dose as most of the beam is absorbed by the patient. Approximate imaging plate:entrance dose ratios are – posteroanterior (PA) chest X-ray (CXR) 1:10, skull X-ray 1:100, AP pelvis 1:1000, lateral lumbar spine X-ray 1:5000 (the actual exit doses are greater due to scatter; these figures are those you would get when the scatter radiation has been removed by the grid).

2b. False

A beam with a higher kV will be more penetrating which increases the proportion of high energy photons that reach the imaging plate. This means that a lower tube current can be used to achieve a similar degree of film blackening and therefore entrance surface dose will be less.

2c. False

Photons at the low energy end of the spectrum contribute nothing to image formation but are absorbed by the patient. By using a filter these can be removed from the beam. Patient dose is lowered as a result.

2d. True

Increasing the focus–detector distance results in less attenuation between skin surface and the imaging plate. This means proportionately less attenuation according to the inverse square law, i.e. the skin dose can be reduced for the same dose to the detector.

2e. False

An anti-scatter grid is situated between the patient and the film–screen. It absorbs some of the radiation beam and therefore a higher tube current is required to achieve an adequate film exposure. This results in an increased patient dose.

3a. True ***

It may also be expressed as the size of the smallest visible detail in millimetres, which would be the width of one line from each line pair.

3b. False

Spatial resolution is best when imaging high contrast structures.

3c. False

Image quality is a generic term that refers to the accuracy of the image in both contrast and spatial resolutions.

3d. True

The bigger the difference in attenuation within each structure, the more visible is the change in greyscale.

3e. True

In projection imaging such as radiography and fluoroscopy, the contrast will increase with a greater thickness of the organ, as more of the difference of attenuation of the beam will be due to the organ of interest. It is decreased by a greater thickness of overlying soft tissue as this will average out the difference of the beam attenuated by the organ. In CT the contrast is essentially independent of the overlying soft tissue.

4a. False ***

Increasing the focus–film distance makes the beam more parallel thereby reducing distortion.

4b. False

Geometrical unsharpness is caused by the penumbra effect where X-ray intensity changes gradually across a sharp-edged object. The penumbra occurs because the X-rays do not arise from a true point source, i.e. it is worse with larger focal spots. Round-edged objects cause *absorption* unsharpness.

4c. True

The penumbra effect is also worse with increased object–film distance.

4d. True

This occurs through greater divergence of the transmitted beam.

4e. True

All act to reduce beam divergence.

5a. False ***

Screen unsharpness is unsharpness caused in the screen by spread of light within the phosphorus material. Total unsharpness is approximately $U_t = (U_g^2 + U_m^2 + U_s^2)^{1/2}$.

5b. False

An air gap reduces scatter reaching the film or detector plate, but it increases geometric unsharpness as the photons have further to travel after attenuation within the object and thus can diverge more.

Geometric unsharpness can be reduced by a longer focus to object distance, a shorter object to film distance, and a smaller focal spot.

5c. True

This assumes that the object is travelling at a steady velocity and that the divergence of photons between object and film or detector plate is minimal. Movement unsharpness can be reduced by asking the patient not to move and hold their breath, immobilizing the patient, and using a shorter exposure time.

5d. True

This occurs due to differential photon attenuation across a rounded edge.

5e. True

Exposure times in mammography can be more than one second. One reason for using compression is to limit patient movement.

6a. True ***

The detection of individual photons is a random process. When only very small numbers of photons are detected this statistical difference is a significant proportion of the whole and is represented as variance in the density of the film or the value given to the pixels.

6b. False

Quantum noise is predominant in all X-ray imaging due to the requirement to keep doses as low as is reasonably practicable (ALARP). Electronic noise is predominant in ultrasound.

6c. True

Although with increasing numbers of photons the variation in numbers detected does increase, this variation as a percentage of the total number of events detected decreases. Thus the noise decreases with increasing dose to the patient, or increased efficiency in detecting photons, or thicker phosphor material, etc.

6d. True

SNR increases in proportion to the square root of the number of photons detected.

6e. False

Structural noise is caused by variations in the structure of the screen phosphor. In modern, precisely made phosphors structural noise is negligible.

7a. True ****

Increasing the kV will result in more high energy photons being produced which will result in a more penetrating or 'harder' beam.

7b. False

Focus to film distance has no significant effect on the quality of the beam. Air will very slightly attenuate the beam to make it slightly harder, but at the distances used in radiology this effect is negligible.

7c. True

Increasing the thickness of the aluminium will attenuate more of the lower energy photons; the exiting beam will have higher average photon energy.

7d. False

This will result in more photons, but the photons will still have the same proportion of energies as long as the kV remains the same.

7e. False

Increased thickness of screen will allow more photons to be absorbed thus allowing a reduced dose at the expense of more screen unsharpness and increased noise. It will have no effect on the quality of the beam unless the kV is changed.

8a. False ***

Scatter falls randomly across the entire image increasing the overall level of grey in the picture. This is similar to a film with a higher base fog and reduces the contrast seen in the image. While spatial resolution is affected (especially of low contrast structures) reduction in contrast is far more significant.

8b. False

Increasing the kV may allow a reduction in the patient dose for the same detector, but the beam becomes more penetrating. A greater proportion of the scatter therefore is formed at the exit side of the patient and so more scatter reaches the imaging detector.

8c. True

The grid predominantly absorbs scatter and allows most of the primary beam to pass through. As higher doses are required, however, the amount of scatter formed within the patient is actually increased.

8d. True

As the grid reduces scatter reaching the detector, the contrast resolution will improve.

8e. False

Grids significantly reduce the amount of radiation reaching the detector and therefore require a higher dose.

9a. True ***

Compression reduces the thickness of material through which the beam travels, so reducing the attenuation of the beam.

9b. True

As the beam passes through less tissue there are fewer Compton interaction events and therefore less scatter is produced.

9c. False

Not only is the amount of scatter reduced thus improving contrast, there is less overlying soft tissue above and below the organ or region of interest. The differing attenuation of the organ therefore becomes more pronounced as it is not superimposed by other soft tissues.

9d. False

As attenuation is reduced, exposure settings can either be left unaltered for a better quality of image or be reduced. They do not need to be increased.

9e. False

Compression is commonly used in mammography, but it may also be used in other settings. Intravenous urography (IVU) studies and abdominal radiographs in large patients would both be examples where compression may be useful if there are no contraindications.

10a. True **
The cathode is the filament and the anode contains the target.

10b. False
The electron beam is emitted from the cathode and bombards the anode target to produce X-rays.

10c. False
An increase in angle would result in a larger effective focal spot size.

10d. False
The focusing cup refers to the shaped part of the cathode that focuses the electrons emitted from the filament towards the target.

10e. True
For older single phase generator systems the average kV is lower and heat loading is calculated using $0.7 \times kVp \times mAs$.

11a. True ***
A metal such as silver in powder form may be used. Conventional liquid lubricants would evaporate in a vacuum.

11b. False
Heat loss via conduction occurs in stationary anodes. In rotating anodes a poor heat conductor such as molybdenum is used as the stem to reduce the chance of heat damage to the bearings. Heat is lost via radiation from the blackened disk to oil around the vacuum casing.

11c. False
The anode disk rotates at a fixed speed which may be as fast as 9000 rpm to evenly distribute heating around the track.

11d. False
The disc is bevelled to provide a surface at an angle. The smaller the angle theta the smaller is the effective focal spot size.

11e. True
The smaller size used in mammography allows better resolution in the image.

12a. False ***
Three phase generators produce a higher average kV but the kVp is unaltered.

12b. True
As the average kV is lower in single phase generators, a higher mA or a longer exposure time is required.

12c. True
High frequency generators are used in most modern diagnostic X-ray sets.

12d. False
Self rectifying generators are still commonly used for dental intraoral radiography. They work on the principle that the X-ray tube current can only flow in one direction, and thus for half the exposure time the tube is switched off. This obviously lowers the average kV, and requires significantly longer exposure times.

12e. True
As the kV across the X-ray tube is always within a few percent of the maximum, the peak of the X-ray spectrum will be shifted to the right and the quality of the beam will be more penetrating.

13a. True **

The minimum filtration required is 2.5 mm of aluminium for which the HVL in aluminium is approximately 2.5 mm. At 125 kV the HVL would be much greater at about 4.5 mm.

13b. True

This is a device that estimates kV by measurement of the differential transmission of the beam through different filter thicknesses. A direct reading of kV can be made using a potential divider, but the less invasive and more commonly used method is with a penetrameter.

13c. True

This consists of many circular details of different diameters and thickness.

13d. True

Tears due to the apron being incorrectly stored may show as lines of X-ray exposure on a film or detector plate.

13e. True

Geometrical distortion is easily identified in this manner.

14a. False **

This is a device for measuring optical density of film.

14b. True

Any deviation greater than agreed levels is reported to a manager responsible for remedial action.

14c. True

This is a requirement under Ionising Radiation (Medical Exposure) Regulations (IR(ME)R).

14d. True

This roughly equates to 10% error.

14e. True

Auditing patient dose for a large patient sample in order to reduce the effect of patient-to-patient variation can demonstrate the effects of equipment differences, operator technique, or differences in patient groups (e.g. elderly versus young adult).

15a. True **

Generally the silver halide is approximately 10% bromide and 90% iodide.

15b. False

Single-sided films are used where spatial resolution is paramount such as in mammography. For general radiography there is emulsion on both sides of the base and two intensifying screens are used to maximize sensitivity to X-rays.

15c. False

The emulsion layer would typically be $5-10$ μm thick.

15d. True

Crystal size affects film speed and gamma, but is typically in the region of 1 μm diameter.

15e. False

The silver halide crystals are most responsive to visible light; this is why intensifying screens are used. They are relatively insensitive to X-rays.

16a. True **

A large variation in crystal size results in a low gamma film while a more uniform crystal size results in a high gamma film. A greater average size of crystals results in a faster film.

16b. True

Although at higher temperatures and concentrations the effective gamma may reduce because of the increased film fog.

16c. False

The higher the gamma of the film the more reduced the useful exposure and thus the latitude.

16d. False

Development of the film is by an alkaline reducing agent which reduces the silver bromide crystals that have been affected by exposure to light into grains of metallic silver. Fixing occurs after this and involves an acid solution such as thiosulphate to dissolve out unaffected silver ions so that the film is no longer susceptible to light and radiation.

16e. True

This adds to fog and decreases the contrast of the film.

17a. True ***

Speed of a film–screen combination changes with different factors such as X-ray beam quality, so speed measurements are given for a specific radiation quality.

17b. True

This is calculated as speed = 1000/air kerma.

17c. False

The quantum sink is the part of the process where the image is carried by the least number of photons. It is this phase where the statistical variation in photon absorption and thus noise will be greatest in comparison to the signal. In film–screen radiography, the quantum sink is at the stage of X-ray photon absorption in the phosphor.

17d. False

$OD = \log_{10}$ (incident light/transmitted light).

17e. False

An OD of about 1 is ideal for most areas of interest. The higher the OD the blacker the appearance of the film. An OD of 2 might be seen in imaging of the lung. ODs of greater than 2.5 are normally too dark to discern any detail. Bones appear light with density generally less than 1.

18a. True **

A commonly used example is gadolinium oxysulphide which has a K-edge of around 50 keV.

18b. False

Typically, screens undergo fluorescence with instantaneous release of light with an intensity which is proportional to the X-rays incident on the screen. Thermoluminescence means light is released after heating.

18c. True

In general radiography there is an intensifying screen on either side of the double emulsion film. In mammography where a higher resolution is required, only one screen and corresponding emulsion are used.

18d. False

They are plotted as OD against the *log* of exposure.

18e. True

A steeper slope represents a larger film gamma.

19a. False ***

It should be around 0.15–0.2.

19b. False

A high gamma implies a narrow range of exposures between black and white in the image; this is equivalent to a narrow latitude.

19c. False

The thickness is a compromise between sensitivity and unsharpness. It needs to be thick enough to efficiently absorb X-ray photons. This is balanced against unsharpness, however, since interactions occurring further from the film will lead to greater spread of the produced light.

19d. True

A balance has to be struck; for the same detection efficiency a better phosphor will increase noise, while a thicker one will increase unsharpness without increasing noise. The greater the X-ray to light conversion factor, the lower the number of photons detected to get the same OD. The quantum noise in the image is inversely proportional to the number of photons detected.

19e. False

Crossover refers to light from one screen affecting the opposite emulsion. Parallax means two emulsions produce two slightly different superimposed images; this is impossible therefore with a single emulsion.

20a. True ***

The intensifying screen essentially amplifies the number of photons detected by the film and so produces a much darker image for the same dose. This means that significantly fewer X-ray photons are detected for the same level of OD and therefore the noise is increased.

20b. False

Film alone absorbs only about 2% of X-ray photons.

20c. True

Intensification factor is typically in the range of 30–100.

20d. False

Rare earth elements such as gadolinium actually have lower atomic numbers than tungsten used in traditional screens. The advantage of rare earth screens is a K-edge that is closer to the average energy of diagnostic X-ray spectrums than the K-edge of tungsten. In addition the rare earth phosphors produce greater light output for each X-ray photon detected.

20e. False

A thicker phosphor layer absorbs more photons. As more photons are absorbed, dose can be reduced proportionally so that the same OD can be achieved at a lower dose with no increase in noise. However, light spreads further within the phosphor layer and so screen unsharpness is increased.

21a. True ***
Molybdenum and rhodium are the most common.

21b. False
The K-edge of an element is just higher than its characteristic radiation, therefore any element is relatively transparent to its own characteristic radiation. Mammography exploits this by commonly using molybdenum as both the anode target and the filter. A molybdenum filter should not be used with a rhodium target as the maximum absorption energies in the filter would correspond to the energy of the characteristic radiation from the target.

21c. False
Film mammography does achieve 15 lp/mm. The pixel size in digital radiography systems for mammography is generally not less than about 70 μm corresponding to 7 lp/mm. However, smaller high contrast details (micro-calcifications) may be seen due to the partial volume effect and the other advantages of digital systems, particularly post processing, mean that increasing numbers of hospitals are moving to digital.

21d. True
At a dose of 2 mGy the risk of inducing fatal cancer in the 50–65-year-old age group is 1 in 50 000. In screening programmes the ALARP principle is especially important.

21e. True
Most mammography exposures are at the lower end of this range.

22a. True **
The movement of the plate and tube causes the shadow of objects above and below the selected slice to move across the plate and become blurred, leaving only the image of objects within the selected slice in focus.

22b. True
To adjust the level of the cut plane slice, the pivot height is adjusted up or down.

22c. False
The slice thickness is increased by reducing the angle of movement. If the angle of movement was zero then a conventional radiograph would be taken with all structures within the slice thickness.

22d. False
Zonography uses a small angle to take a thick slice to image an entire organ or when contrast is expected to be low.

22e. True
This blurring combined with increased attenuation of the beam passing obliquely through the patient leads to higher doses being needed compared with a conventional radiograph.

23a. False ****
Dual energy radiography uses a composite of two images obtained with different tube voltages. They can then be subtracted from one another to form an image with high soft tissue contrast (subtract low kV

from high kV) or an image with high bone contrast (subtract high kV from low kV).

23b. True

A low kV beam will have higher contrast.

23c. True

Subtracting the high kV image from the low kV image will improve contrast of the bony structures.

23d. False

Subtraction of the high kV image from the low kV image will improve detection of calcified structures

23e. False

Contrast enhanced angiography uses a digital subtraction technique, where the pre-injection image is subtracted from the post-injection image to show only the contrast filled vessels. DSA stands for digital subtraction angiography.

4. Digital Radiography: Questions

1. Digital imaging:
   a. Pixel size, field of view and matrix size (number of pixels) are inter-related
   b. Spatial resolution is not related to pixel size
   c. A 12-bit pixel depth means there are 12^2 (144) levels of grey
   d. A greater bit depth is required for plain film radiography compared with nuclear medical imaging
   e. Compression of data can reduce storage space by up to 40 times

2. Image processing:
   a. In digital imaging, the image is divided into a matrix of pixels each with a greyscale value attached to it
   b. Digital images may be easily adjusted post acquisition to correct for overexposure or underexposure
   c. Detector dose indicators (DDIs) are measurements provided to indicate the level of exposure of the radiograph
   d. Algorithms for edge enhancement or noise reduction may be applied to increase image quality
   e. Images of chest and abdominal radiographs are typically about 1024×768 pixels

3. Computed radiography:
   a. Computed radiography uses a thermoluminescent phosphor imaging plate
   b. The imaging plate is read by a laser scanning across the plate to release light proportional to the X-ray photons absorbed by each part of the plate
   c. The laser light used is a different frequency to the light emitted by the plate
   d. Scanning time for a photostimulable plate is typically in the region of 30 sec
   e. Computed radiography has an improved contrast and spatial resolution compared to film–screen systems

4. Digital radiography:
   a. The detector plate acquires a digital image without having to be physically taken to a scanner
   b. Digital detector plates are fragile and only used in fixed locations such as table and wall Bucky systems
   c. Direct digital radiography systems use amorphous silicon thin film transistor (TFT) arrays
   d. Indirect systems use a phosphor to absorb X-rays and release light photons which produce the image
   e. Digital radiography is more expensive than computed radiography

5. Fourier analysis:

a. Fourier analysis involves transforming a signal into a series of sine waves

b. Fourier analysis of one term is equivalent to an exact reproduction of even a complicated image

c. The Nyquist criterion states that the signal must be sampled at least once in every period to avoid the possibility of aliasing

d. The Nyquist frequency is half the sampling frequency

e. Fourier analysis is used exclusively in computed radiography to convert the analogue image from the phosphor into binary data

6. Modulation transfer function (MTF):

a. MTF is a measure of how well an image represents the original object

b. MTF reduces at higher object spatial frequencies

c. The MTF is equal to 1/line spread function (LSF)

d. The total MTF is the product of the MTFs of all the constituent parts of the imaging system

e. The MTF of a perfect system would be 1

7. PACS:

a. Stands for patient archived computed system

b. Allows simultaneous reading of an image by many users

c. Stores all of the images locally on each viewing terminal in the department

d. A PACS broker sells the necessary software

e. Images are stored as JPEGs

4. Digital Radiography: Answers

1a. True **
Pixel size = field of view (FOV)/matrix size.

1b. False
In theory, the smallest detail resolvable is equal to pixel size although smaller high contrast detail, e.g. microcalcification, may be visible due to the partial volume effect.

1c. False
A bit depth of 12 means there are 2^{12} (4096) levels of grey.

1d. True
Plain film radiography has a large dynamic range; this requires a large bit depth. Bit depth in nuclear medical imaging relates to counts per pixel; numerically, these counts are smaller than the dynamic range of plain film radiography.

1e. True
Lossless compression can reduce the size of a file by 2–3 times; this is fully reversible. Lossy compression is not fully reversible but provides an order of magnitude more compression.

2a. True ***
This matrix may then be used to display the picture on a monitor.

2b. True
This reduces the number of repeat films that have to be taken. Although an image that was underexposed can still be adjusted in this way, the low signal to noise ratio (SNR) may cause the radiograph to appear unacceptably grainy.

2c. True
As digital radiographs that have been overexposed will be automatically adjusted to look as though taken at the perfect exposure, higher doses may be given without the operator necessarily appreciating this. The DDI for an image may be compared to an expected range of values to show whether or not the image was correctly exposed. This helps to ensure that the principle of keeping doses as low as is reasonably practicable (ALARP) is being observed.

2d. True
These techniques use the signal from adjacent pixels to either average the signal reducing noise but blurring the image slightly or to enhance the contrast at a structure edge at the expense of increasing noise and possibly creating false detail.

2e. False
Large plates used for chest and abdominal radiographs are typically in the region of 2500 × 3000 pixels (7.5 megapixels). Smaller plates may be about 2000 × 2500 (5 megapixels) but with each pixel being smaller to improve spatial resolution.

3a. False **

A photostimulable phosphor is used, commonly a barium fluorohalide.

3b. True

This released light is collected using a network of optical fibres and amplified and detected by a photomultiplier tube.

3c. True

This helps minimize laser light being reflected and being included in the final image. Most computed radiography phosphors emit blue light and the plate is scanned with a red light laser.

3d. True

To maximize throughput in a busy department stacking readers are used to automatically place plates in a queue so radiographers do not have to spend additional time manually loading each cassette.

3e. False

While the dynamic range and thus the possible contrast are significantly improved, computed radiography has a poorer spatial resolution when compared with film–screen systems. This is primarily due to the larger pixel size and light spread within the phosphor during reading.

4a. True *

This allows fast throughput of patients, especially for quick examinations such as outpatient chest X-ray (CXR).

4b. False

This may be true for certain types of detector, but indirect digital radiography detectors using non-crystalline phosphors such as gadolinium oxysulphide are more robust and can be used in alternative positions including for ward radiography and may have wireless connections for PACS.

4c. False

Amorphous silicon is used for light detection from a phosphor such as caesium iodide (CsI). Amorphous selenium is used to allow the direct conversion of the X-ray photons to a charge captured by the TFT array.

4d. True

These systems commonly use a phosphor layer such as CsI to convert X-rays into light before capturing the light photons via photodiodes in a TFT array or via tiled charge coupled device (CCD) detectors.

4e. True

Computed radiography cassettes can be used with the same Bucky tables and X-ray tubes, only requiring a reader to be installed in the department which may service several rooms. Digital radiography systems require a separate detector, or sometimes even more than one detector per room, each of which is very expensive.

5a. True ****

The signal is interpreted as a series of sine waves with variable magnitude that when added together reproduce the original signal.

5b. False

The more terms (additional sine waves at multiples of the original frequency) the closer the composite signal is to the original. An infinite number of terms would produce a perfect copy of the original signal.

5c. False

The Nyquist criterion states that the signal must be sampled at least twice in every period to avoid the possibility of aliasing.

5d. True

The Nyquist frequency is the maximum frequency that can be sampled without aliasing. Because the signal needs to be sampled twice in every period, the maximum frequency that can be sampled accurately is half the sampling frequency.

5e. False

Fourier analysis is also used for reconstruction of tomographic images in, for example, computed tomography (CT) and magnetic resonance imaging (MRI).

6a. True *****

MTF ranges from 0–100%. Low spatial frequencies are generally well represented by an imaging system (near 100%); as this frequency goes up, the MTF goes down.

6b. True

The MTF is dependent on the spatial frequency of the object. Whilst even a simple system could image a series of thick lines spaced 2 cm apart each with almost perfect accuracy, even modern complicated radiology systems cannot accurately image lines spaced a few micro-metres apart.

6c. False

The LSF is calculated from the unsharpness of the boundary between a region of very high and very low contrast (an edge). The MTF is calculated from LSF using Fourier transform analysis.

6d. True

Knowing the MTF of each constituent part allows the MTF of different film–screen combinations to be predicted.

6e. True

In a perfect imaging system the MTF would be 1 and would not change with object spatial frequency.

7a. False ***

Picture Archiving and Communication System.

7b. True

This is one of the benefits of PACS: radiographs can be viewed on the ward at the same time as being reported by the radiology department. Also, old radiographs are instantly available.

7c. False

Hence the term *archive*. Images are stored centrally on servers.

7d. False

The broker is simply further software that allows *communication* between the different information systems within the hospital thus integrating the various electronic records.

7e. False

Images are stored as Digital Imaging and Communications in Medicine (DICOM) files. A DICOM image file also contains data about the patient, display preferences and imaging modality.

5. Fluoroscopy: Questions

1. Structure of the image intensifier:
   a. The input screen is always larger than the output screen
   b. The input screen is normally made from caesium iodide (CsI) crystals
   c. The input screen detects approximately 60% of the incoming X-ray photons
   d. The photocathode is attached to the output screen
   e. The potential difference across the intensifier of about 25 kV accelerates electrons towards the photocathode

2. More structure of the image intensifier:
   a. The output screen is normally about 15–40 cm in diameter
   b. A layer of aluminium is placed over the inner surface of the output phosphor to improve its mechanical strength
   c. Focusing electrodes use positive potentials to concentrate the path of the electron beam
   d. One of the functions of the intensifier housing is to prevent light from entering the intensifier
   e. The output screen is normally made of sodium iodide (NaI)

3. Gain and magnification:
   a. Gain is the ratio of the brightness of the output phosphor over that of the input phosphor
   b. Overall gain is the sum of the flux gain and the minification gain
   c. An increase in gain increases the signal to noise ratio (SNR)
   d. By changing the voltages on the focusing electrodes the focal electron crossover point is moved closer to the input screen to magnify the image
   e. Magnification uses a smaller area of the output screen to increase the minification gain

4. Automatic brightness control and dose control curves:
   a. Automatic brightness control adjusts the gain automatically to keep the monitor image at the same level of brightness
   b. Automatic brightness control is normally set by the brightness at the centre of the image or the set region of interest
   c. Dose control curves always increase kV in preference to mA to keep patient dose as low as is reasonably practicable (ALARP)
   d. Dose control curves can be selected by the operator depending on the quality of image required
   e. Modern image intensifiers use charge coupled device (CCD) cameras to acquire the image displayed on the output phosphor

5. **Dose rates and usual doses for fluoroscopy:**
   a. Skin entrance dose rates should never exceed 100 mGy per minute
   b. Dose is generally higher for pulsed fluoroscopy than for continuous fluoroscopy
   c. A typical effective dose for a barium meal would be 2.5 mSv
   d. A typical equivalent dose for a barium enema would be 7 mSv
   e. Screening times for a barium enema are typically in the range of 1–3 min

6. **Safety in fluoroscopy screening:**
   a. Staff members who do not have to be next to the patient should stand back to take advantage of the inverse square law
   b. Under couch tubes result in more radiation exposure to an operator standing next to the patient than over couch tubes
   c. Most scatter is from the point where the beam exits the patient
   d. The lead shielding around the intensifier provides adequate protection from the primary beam
   e. A lead apron combined with a thyroid shield provides adequate protection from the primary beam

7. **Image quality and noise in image intensifiers:**
   a. Noise in fluoroscopy is predominantly electrical noise caused by minification gain
   b. SNR can be increased by increasing the kV across the intensifier
   c. SNR can be increased by frame averaging
   d. Typical resolution on the monitor of a fluoroscopy system is 1.2–3 lp/mm depending on magnification
   e. Veiling glare and geometrical distortion are common artefacts in fluoroscopy

8. **In traditional fluoroscopic image intensifiers:**
   a. Brightness gain increases with increasing voltage across the intensifier
   b. Brightness gain increases with the use of magnification
   c. Brightness gain is increased when the exposure to the input phosphor is increased
   d. Vignetting causes the periphery of the image to be brighter than the centre
   e. Geometrical distortion may cause the periphery of the image to be distorted

9. **Digital subtraction angiography (DSA):**
   a. A mask image for the subtraction needs to be taken after injection of contrast
   b. DSA cannot be viewed in realtime because the images need to be processed in the computer before the subtracted image can be displayed
   c. Slight movements between the mask and subtracted images may produce dark or light lines along high contrast structures such as bones
   d. DSA requires at least two frames per second to image arteries, with slower frame rates being used for venous structures
   e. Subtracted images have a decreased SNR

10. **Flat plate detectors:**
    a. Contrast using a flat plate detector is much better than traditional fluoroscopy
    b. Flat plate detectors do not suffer from veiling glare or geometric distortion
    c. Spatial resolution is not as good using digital flat plate detectors when compared with traditional fluoroscopy
    d. Flat plate X-ray photon detection efficiency is comparable to traditional fluoroscopy
    e. Flat plate detectors can be made much smaller compared with image intensifier explorators

5. Fluoroscopy: Answers

1a. True ***

This size difference contributes towards the intensification via minification gain.

1b. True

Caesium (K-edge 36 keV) and iodine (K-edge 33 keV) are very effective at detecting X-ray photons at the peak of the Bremsstrahlung peak of most fluoroscopic examinations. These K-edges are also very similar to those of commonly used contrast agents for most screening procedures.

1c. True

CsI is arranged in thin crystals that internally reflect light photons. This helps prevent light spread allowing a thicker layer of phosphor (0.1–0.4 mm) to be used where more photons can be detected without increasing screen unsharpness to an unacceptable level.

1d. False

The photocathode is attached to the input screen and releases electrons when hit by photons from the phosphor.

1e. False

The potential difference is commonly about 25 kV, but this accelerates electrons away from the negative photocathode towards the positively charged anode at the output screen.

2a. False ***

The input screen is about 15–40 cm diameter. The output screen diameter is between about 20 and 35 mm.

2b. False

The thin aluminium layer prevents light emitted back from the output phosphor being detected by the photocathode. This feedback would cause complete 'white-out' of the image.

2c. True

The electrodes control the voltage gradient across the tube and ensure that they are focused onto the output screen. They act like an electron lens.

2d. True

Other functions are to maintain the vacuum within the intensifier and to shield from magnetic fields. Lead shielding is also normally placed around the unit to protect the operator.

2e. False

The output screen is normally made of zinc cadmium sulphide. NaI crystals are commonly used in gamma cameras.

3a. True ***

Gain is not normally measured, however, as it is difficult to measure the brightness of the input phosphor. Conversion factor (G_x) is used instead, which is the ratio of the brightness of the output phosphor and the dose rate of X-rays at the input phosphor.

3b. False

Overall gain is the product of the flux gain and the minification gain. As flux gain is typically about 50, and minification gain typically about 100 when not using magnification settings, a typical overall gain would be 5000.

3c. False

The quantum sink is the detection of X-ray photons at the phosphor. Gain will multiply the signal, but will also multiply the noise equally. A greater gain would also allow a lower dose to be used to achieve the same brightness on the monitor, and if a lower dose is used a decrease in the SNR would be observed.

3d. True

This results in a smaller section of the input screen being used and therefore the minification gain decreases, but the image of the region viewed is magnified.

3e. False

Using a smaller area of the output screen would increase the minification gain but would not result in a magnified image.

4a. False ***

Automatic brightness control adjusts the kV and/or mA to keep the image brightness constant. The gain is kept constant unless magnification is used.

4b. True

Many systems are just set to the centre of the image, but intensifier systems may have more complicated regions of interest set, or may allow the regions of interest to be customized. In almost all cases the brightness at the periphery of the image is ignored, which means that lung or air to the side of the patient does not overly affect the image.

4c. False

Some dose control curves are set this way, and minimize dose but at the expense of image quality. Other dose control curves predominantly increase mA and keep kV fairly constant, which may be used when the kV is optimized for the K-edge of a particular contrast agent. Most dose control curves increase kV and mA together.

4d. True

Many systems allow the user to select the appropriate dose control curve for the type of examination. This allows a higher quality but higher dose control curve when needed or a low quality low dose when high contrast and resolution diagnostic images are not required, such as in placement of a nasogastric tube.

4e. True

Older intensifiers used vacuum device video cameras. CCDs produce a direct digital signal. They have a better resolution with a 1024 × 1024 or higher display. They can provide digital feedback for the automatic brightness control system instead of requiring a partially reflecting mirror for older optical cameras.

5a. True **

Remedial action is required if entrance dose rates exceed 50 mGy/min for the largest field size. Typical dose rates are in the region of 10–30 mGy/min.

5b. False

Pulsed fluoroscopy works with short bursts of radiation, often set at about 3 pulses per second, to give an image. Although this can result in blurring if there is any movement, for many screening procedures such as barium enemas this is quite acceptable. As the X-ray tube is only on intermittently, the dose over time falls approximately proportionate to the pulse rate.

5c. True

This is roughly equivalent to a year of average background radiation in the UK.

5d. False

A typical effective dose would be 7 mSv.

5e. True

Screening times for different studies can vary quite widely depending on the patient and operator, but this range would be typical.

6a. True **

Helper staff or nurses from the ward may not be aware of radiation protection issues and should be guided as to where to stand. Although the patient is not a point source, the inverse square law is still a good rough estimation and shows that increased distance from the patient significantly reduces exposure to scattered radiation.

6b. False

Over couch tube systems typically expose an operator standing near the patient to more scattered radiation.

6c. False

Most scatter is from the point where the primary beam enters the patient, as here the beam is not yet attenuated by the patient and is far more intense.

6d. True

The lead shielding of the intensifier is typically 2 mm or more and effectively stops the primary beam.

6e. False

Lead aprons are only commonly made up to 0.5 mm lead equivalence, and most are 0.35 mm. This provides adequate protection from scattered radiation for the body parts covered, but not from the primary beam.

7a. False **

As with other X-ray radiography, the requirement to keep doses ALARP means that the number of absorbed X-ray photons is the quantum sink, and that quantum mottle is the predominant cause of noise in the image.

7b. False

Increasing kV across the intensifier would increase flux gain, but this would increase noise in the same proportion and therefore the SNR would not change.

7c. True

Frame averaging adds the signal from successive frames taken over a period of time. This increases the SNR and provides a higher quality image as long as the patient does not move during this time.

7d. True

The resolutions of the television and display systems are the limiting factors.

7e. True

Veiling glare is caused by light scattering within the output phosphor and results in loss of contrast in darker areas. It also results in the centre of the image being brighter than the periphery. Geometrical distortion is caused by focusing inaccuracies and by the curved input screen that tends to magnify the periphery of the image. This is not normally noticeable when imaging the complex organs of the body, but images of straight objects such as wires in interventional work may be noticeably bent by this effect.

8a. True ***

The electron emitted from the input screen is accelerated by the voltage to the output screen, gaining energy as it does so. The greater the voltage, the greater the energy gained and the more photons emitted from the output screen; this is flux gain.

8b. False

Magnification uses a smaller area of the input screen focused on the same area of output screen. The minification gain is therefore less.

8c. False

Brightness gain is the multiplication factor the intensifier has increased the original signal by. Increasing the original signal does not affect this.

8d. False

Vignetting is caused by light spread in both the output and input phosphors and with electron spread within the intensifier. It causes the central area to be brighter than the periphery and reduces contrast.

8e. True

The periphery of the image is magnified slightly more than the centre due to the curve of the input screen, and S-type distortion can occur from small changes in the magnetic fields influencing the paths of the electrons.

9a. False **

The mask image is of normal anatomy to be subtracted from the later images with contrast to leave only an image of contrast within the vessels. Therefore the mask image needs to be taken prior to contrast reaching the vessels.

9b. False

Modern computers are easily able to handle this in fractions of a second and display a subtracted image with no perceptible delay. More advanced techniques such as pixel shift to improve the image from minor movements may be done after the sequence is acquired, but a simple realtime image is displayed immediately.

9c. True

This may be cancelled to some extent by pixel shift techniques. Excessive movement will make interpretation of structures more difficult, as lines along the edges of bones may obscure vessels.

9d. False

While high frame rates may be required for large arteries such as the aorta and iliac vessels, peripheral arteries such as the lower limb arteries would commonly be imaged at 1 frame per second.

9e. True

This essentially works in the opposite way to frame averaging and may require a higher dose when compared with non-subtracted imaging.

10a. True **

The dynamic range of conventional fluoroscopy is normally no greater than 30:1. Digital flat plate detectors are capable of 14 bit depth (i.e. 16 000 level of grey). The full range is not required allowing images at much higher or lower dose levels.

10b. True

Light spread within the flat plate CsI crystals is significantly less than the veiling glare of the output phosphor of traditional fluoroscopy. Flat plate detectors image in the same way that digital radiography systems do and therefore there is no curved input plate or focusing of electron beams to distort the image.

10c. False

Flat plate detectors can have resolutions at 3 lp/mm or more, and this resolution is irrespective of magnification. This compares favourably even to the resolution of the highest magnifications of traditional fluoroscopy and is much better than the 1.2 lp/mm of unmagnified fluoroscopy.

10d. True

Both flat plate and traditional fluoroscopy systems detect about 60–65% of X-ray photons.

10e. True

The flat plate system does not have to contain the bulky vacuum intensifier. The unit still has to be connected to an X-ray tube, however, and the lead shielding is still very heavy. Nevertheless, the appearance may be far less concerning to claustrophobic patients.

1. **Computed tomography (CT) image reconstruction and basics:**
   a. CT images are formed from a matrix of voxels each with an assigned number representing the X-ray attenuation coefficient of a corresponding volume within the patient
   b. Filtered back projection is a process in which the number assigned to each voxel from each projection is adjusted by a function of the measured amounts in the neighbouring pencil beams
   c. Each voxel is measured independently by a pencil beam falling on a particular detector
   d. CT has a higher spatial resolution than conventional plain film radiography
   e. CT has a better contrast resolution than conventional plain film radiography

2. **Image formation in CT:**
   a. The detectors sample a continuously produced X-ray beam approximately 360 times per rotation
   b. Each voxel in a particular image slice is represented by a single detector in the array
   c. The log of the ratio of the unattenuated beam to that detected is equal to the sum of linear attenuation coefficients of each voxel the beam passes through
   d. CT requires higher doses compared with conventional radiography since the beam suffers more attenuation for the same projection
   e. Scout views (survey radiographs) are produced line by line at a fixed projection angle e.g. anteroposterior (AP)

3. **Image reconstruction in CT:**
   a. Utilizes iterative processes
   b. With an infinite number of samples an object could be perfectly reproduced
   c. With back projection each object in the scanner field contributes to every voxel in that image slice
   d. Filtered back projection convolves the image profile
   e. An edge enhancing convolution kernel will reduce spatial resolution

4. Regarding CT images:
a. The effect of quantum noise in an image is reduced by narrowing the viewing window
b. Spatial resolution in the z-direction is unaffected by pitch
c. A CT image is most commonly calculated on a 256×256 matrix
d. Scanned projection radiographs are performed to allow planning of the CT sequence
e. Signal to noise ratio (SNR) is increased by reducing the mAs but keeping the kV constant

5. Ranges of Hounsfield unit (HU) and window settings:
a. The CT number or HU for air is 0
b. The normal HU range for fat is −60 to −150
c. The normal HU range for muscle is 40 to 60
d. Soft tissue window settings might include a window width of 400 and window centre of 30 HU
e. Lung window settings might be: window width 1500 and window centre −600 HU

6. Regarding CT images:
a. CT angiography can utilize maximum intensity projection (MIP) to enhance image quality
b. A structure with an average CT number of −60 is likely to be made up predominantly of muscle
c. For a given kV and mAs, the quantum noise in an image is increased as the field of view (FOV) increases
d. With modern CT equipment, each scan can produce several gigabytes (GB) of data
e. Filtered back projection is not required in image reconstruction when using multi-slice detectors

7. CT gantry and scanner generations:
a. Modern multi-slice CT scanners are examples of 3rd generation scanners
b. 4th generation scanners are the future of advanced CT technology
c. Multi-slice scanners with an excess of 256 detector rows are unlikely to be produced
d. The tube and detector array rotate at approximately 60 revolutions per second in modern CT scanners
e. Spiral CT scans are outdated and no longer commonly used

8. **CT X-ray tubes:**
   a. The CT tube is mounted with its anode–cathode axis perpendicular to the axis of rotation of the scanner to minimize the heel effect
   b. Allow continuous scanning for up to 5 min
   c. CT tubes typically use a focal spot size of approximately 0.6–1 mm
   d. The anode target material used in CT is rhodium because of its higher energy characteristic radiation
   e. CT anodes may require heat capacities of 4 MJ or more and typically require active cooling mechanisms

9. **Collimation and filtration in CT:**
   a. Filtration in CT is typically 2.5 mm equivalent of aluminium
   b. Bow tie filters are used to minimize variance in beam hardening caused by the elliptical shape of the patient
   c. To produce thin 0.5 mm slice in multi-slice CT scanners the collimation is set to just a single row of detectors within the array
   d. Post-patient collimation is essential in multi-slice CT to reduce scatter
   e. The width of the collimation at the level of the axis is typically about 50 cm

10. **CT detector technology:**
    a. Xenon filled ionization chambers are used in most modern multi-slice CT scanners
    b. Solid-state detectors are formed from a scintillant such as cadmium tungstate and a silicon photodiode
    c. Should have negligible afterglow
    d. Separation of detectors to prevent light crossover increases the detection efficiency of the array
    e. Solid-state detectors can be produced to a width of approximately 0.5 mm

11. **Scan parameters in CT:**
    a. A pitch of 1 indicates a contiguous data-set
    b. Settings of 120 kV and 140 mA might be used
    c. Are unchanged when scanning adults and children
    d. Matrix size can be reduced to 256×256 in CT fluoroscopy to enable realtime reconstruction of images
    e. A pitch of 3 is often used to enable scanning the thorax of a patient in a single breath hold

12. Regarding spiral and multi-slice CT:
a. True spiral CT was not possible before the advent of slip ring technology
b. Means that several parallel beams are used in data acquisition
c. The number of slices a scanner is capable of producing per gantry revolution is determined by the number of detector rows
d. Slice width is determined by collimation
e. Beam divergence in the z-axis is a potential problem

13. Noise in CT:
a. Noise limits CT as it reduces contrast and limits the spatial resolution of small low contrast objects
b. Quantum noise is the most significant type in CT
c. SNR may be improved by increasing the mA or the scan time per rotation
d. SNR may be improved by decreasing the slice width on a multi-slice scanner
e. If the mA is kept constant, increasing the kV will increase the SNR

14. Multi-planar reconstruction (MPR) and isotropic voxels:
a. Isotropic voxels describe any cuboidal-shaped voxel
b. Axial CT images acquired using most modern scanners can be reformatted to coronal and sagittal images without losing any data quality
c. MPR techniques can allow oblique sections to obtain true coronal and sagittal images even if the patient was rotated in the scanner
d. The isotropic voxel can be used to create a three-dimensional (3D) data map
e. MIP images are often used to look at the bronchial tree

15. Artefacts in CT:
a. Photon starvation occurs in obese patients
b. Beam hardening artefact means CT numbers in the core of the patient tend to be higher than they should be
c. A ring artefact can occur if a single detector is faulty
d. Partial voluming can potentially make very small highly dense objects appear larger
e. Cone beam artefact does not occur for objects situated close to the centre of rotation of a multi-slice scanner

16. Image artefacts:
a. Photon starvation can be seen as a dark ring starved of photons by a detector fault
b. Slice misregistration can be minimized with spiral scanning techniques
c. Motion artefacts may occur even on rapid spiral CT techniques
d. Streak artefacts rarely cause any significant degradation of the image in modern scanners due to metal correction algorithms
e. Very small high density lesions may appear to have an inaccurately low CT number

17. Dose in CT:
    a. Multi-slice always requires more dose than single slice
    b. Pitch is inversely proportional to dose in CT
    c. The CT Dose Index (CTDI) is a measure of dose in a single rotation of the gantry
    d. In spiral CT, thinner slices lead to an increased dose for the same scanned volume
    e. Automated modulation of the kV compensates for patient size so that variation in dose to the detector is small and therefore quantum mottle remains similar for all patients

18. Regarding CT dose:
    a. CTDI is routinely measured using a thermoluminescent detector
    b. The effective dose from a CT of the abdomen and pelvis approximates 10 mSv
    c. The effective dose from a CT kidneys, ureters and bladder (CT KUB) is 20 times greater than that from an X-ray intravenous urography (IVU)
    d. By using a 64-slice scanner as opposed to a single-slice scanner to image a set volume with identical tube voltage/current, the patient dose is approximately doubled
    e. The centre of the patient receives the highest dose when using a helical scanner

19. Dose in CT:
    a. CT accounts for only 4% of examinations using ionizing radiation, yet accounts for 40% of the total dose
    b. The CTDI gives a value of the total effective dose of the scan
    c. Dose length product (DLP) is the dose of the scan multiplied by the length of the scan in seconds
    d. The effective dose of a CT head is approximately 2 mSv
    e. The effective dose of a CT chest is approximately 8 mSv

20. Contrast and special uses of CT:
    a. The high kV and dose from CT makes it unsuitable for interventional work
    b. Contrast should be given with caution or avoided altogether in patients with poor kidney function
    c. A trained health-care professional must be available at all times when contrast is being administered because of the 1% risk of inducing an anaphylactic reaction
    d. Treatment for anaphylactic reaction may involve intramuscular adrenaline, coticosteroids and antihistamines
    e. Modern CT cardiography can scan the entire heart in less than half a second and thus minimize cardiac motion artefacts

6. Computed Tomography: Answers

1a. True **

Voxels are represented as pixels with a greyscale which corresponds to the calculated density or CT number.

1b. True

This allows a more accurate image reconstruction with less blurring at object edges.

1c. False

There is no known way of measuring each voxel independently. Each pencil beam (the part of the beam falling on one particular detector) at each angle measures the total attenuation of all the voxels it has passed through. When this information from many different angles has been analysed using complex algorithms, the attenuation coefficient for each particular voxel can be calculated.

1d. False

Resolution of CT is limited to approximately 0.5 mm or 1 lp/mm. Conventional film radiography is commonly able to produce 8 lp/mm while digital radiography can achieve 3.5 lp/mm.

1e. True

In a CT slice the depth of tissue displayed corresponds to the slice thickness which is never more than 10 mm and with multidetector computed tomography (MDCT) is commonly no more than 2 mm whereas in conventional radiography the depth is the overall thickness of the patient which may be 200 mm or greater. The overlying structures in conventional radiography significantly reduce the potential for contrast resolution.

2a. False **

The continuous beam is sampled approximately 1000 times per rotation.

2b. False

Each voxel is reconstructed from all projections in the rotation and from many detectors in the array.

2c. True

These multiple overlapping samples are used to calculate the linear attenuation and hence the CT value for each individual voxel.

2d. False

CT requires higher doses since the patient is sampled from multiple directions rather than just one; the extent of attenuation is the same for a given projection.

2e. True

These appear more like standard radiographic images.

3a. False ***

Modern scanners use back projection.

3b. True

This is the mathematical theory described by Radon in 1917 upon which CT reconstruction is based.

3c. True
This creates a blurred image, hence the need for filtering using the convolution kernel.
3d. True
This is a high pass filtering procedure.
3e. False
Edge enhancement increases the differences between neighbouring voxels thereby increasing spatial resolution; this also increases noise.

4a. False **
Noise is more perceptible with a narrower window width but contrast to noise ratio remains the same.
4b. False
Spatial resolution in the z-direction is reduced as pitch increases. This is because a greater degree of interpolation is required to form the image, reducing spatial resolution.
4c. False
Typically 512×512 but larger matrix sizes are being developed.
4d. True
That is the purpose of scanned projection radiographs.
4e. False
Reducing the number of photons forming the image would reduce SNR.

5a. False ***
The HU for water is defined as 0. The HU for air is -1000. Air and water are defined points in the CT number or HU system and are used for calibration of the scanner.
5b. True
Because fat is of lower density than water.
5c. True
Most normal soft tissues are of similar density within a narrow range of values.
5d. True
This gives a good range across the HU for fat, muscle and most organs, while the lungs and bone are poorly imaged as their HUs are outside this range.
5e. True
Lung window settings are centred very much lower as the HU for lung is -300 to -800 and the HU for air is -1000.

6a. True ***
Displaying only the voxels in an image which contain the highest CT number has the effect of 'subtracting' the surrounding structures from a contrast enhanced blood vessel.
6b. False
Muscle typically has a CT number of $+40$ to $+60$. Structures which have a negative CT number would most likely contain fat or gas.

6c. False

With a larger FOV the voxel size is increased. There are therefore more photons passing through each voxel and noise is subsequently decreased.

6d. True

With between 10 and 100 MBs per slice on a 512 × 512 matrix, large volumes of data can quickly be produced.

6e. False

Filtered back projection is fundamental in all CT image reconstruction.

7a. True *

All multi-slice scanners utilize a rotate–rotate 3rd generation type of scanner, where both the tube and detector array rotate around the patient.

7b. False

The generation system of describing scanners does not mean that the higher the generation number the more advanced the scanner. 4th generation may have been appropriate to single-slice scanning but for multi-slice, which is now standard, 3rd generation geometry is the norm.

7c. False

Multi-slice scanners with 320 rows of detectors are already being produced.

7d. False

A maximum of 2 to 4 revolutions per second can be achieved with a modern CT scanner.

7e. False

Modern CT scanners acquire images in a spiral or helical fashion.

8a. False **

A CT X-ray tube is mounted parallel to the axis of the scanner for this reason.

8b. False

Due to considerable heat loading from the high voltages used, continuous scanning is limited to around 90 sec. This is enough to allow large volumes to be scanned in a single pass and very much greater than is needed for standard examination particularly with 64-slice equipment.

8c. True

There are often two focal spots available depending on application.

8d. False

Rhodium and molybdenum are used in mammography for their characteristic radiation. CT typically uses tungsten for the same reasons as plain film radiography.

8e. True

A typical individual CT scan may require the tube to be operated at 120 kV and 200 mA for up to 90 sec, producing a significant amount of heat in the tube. Active heat exchangers allow this heat to be removed from the oil around the tube more quickly and reduce the chance of overheating.

9a. False ***
This would be typical of plain film radiography. CT typically uses about 6 mm of aluminium or other materials such as copper.

9b. True
This also reduces an unnecessarily large dose to the periphery of the patient that is generally thinner than at the centre.

9c. False
It is not necessary to do this. The collimation is normally kept set to the entire detector array and the single slice is reconstructed from the data obtained by the 0.5 mm wide detectors.

9d. False
Post-patient collimation was sometimes used in single detector row scanners. In modern multi-slice detectors, however, post-patient collimation would also shield the other detectors from the main beam and is therefore not used. Reasonable scatter reduction is achieved in the air gap between the patient and detector array.

9e. True
This is of sufficient size to scan most patients.

10a. False ***
Xenon ionization chambers cannot be used in multi-slice scanners and have been replaced by solid-state detectors

10b. True
Other scintillants commonly used include rare earth ceramics or bismuth germanate.

10c. True
They also need to have a high detection efficiency, fast response, wide dynamic range and a stable, noise-free response. Solid-state detectors can fulfil all these criteria.

10d. False
The scintillant materials of the detectors have to be separated by an opaque material to prevent light crossover; however, this reduces the overall detection efficiency from 98% to approximately 80%.

10e. True
The size of the individual detectors limits the smallest size of the voxel produced in the image, currently about 0.5 mm in width.

11a. True *
A pitch of 1 means that the table movement equals the combined width of the active detectors and therefore the data-set is contiguous.

11b. True
Tube voltage is usually set between 80 and 140 kV; current often ranges from 100 to 200 mA.

11c. False
The effective dose received can be four times greater in children if adult scan parameters are used; clinically therefore, paediatric scanning uses less current.

11d. True

Standard CT imaging uses a 512 × 512 matrix, but other sizes can be used.

11e. False

For accurate reconstruction, pitch is usually set between 1 and 2.

12a. True ***

Continuous acquisition of a spiral data-set requires an uninhibited gantry rotation.

12b. False

One beam is used; rather there are multiple rows of detectors.

12c. False

Commonly there are more detector rows than slices produced at any one time; this allows varying combinations of slice thickness. The slice number that defines the scanner is based on the maximum number of active data channels at any given time.

12d. False

The total beam width is determined by collimation; it is not possible to collimate each slice, active detector width determines slice thickness in multi-slice scanning.

12e. True

Generally when there are more than four slices the beam is considered to be divergent in the z-axis; this is known as a cone beam. If there are less than four slices, then z-axis divergence is not as important; fan beam geometry is assumed. Cone beam geometry has implications for image artefacts.

13a. True ***

As with conventional radiology, image quality is constantly balanced against keeping ionizing radiation as low as is reasonably practicable (ALARP).

13b. True

There is also structural and electronic noise. Quantum is more common due to the relatively low doses used.

13c. True

This is at the expense of an increased dose to the patient.

13d. False

If the other parameters are kept the same, a thinner slice width will decrease the number of photons falling on that particular width, and therefore decrease the SNR. In MPR, however, several layers can be added together post-processing to increase the SNR again at the expense of a thicker slice, and so data are commonly acquired at the thinnest slice possible even if it will eventually be viewed as thicker slices.

13e. True

Increasing the kV will make the beam harder, fewer photons will be absorbed by the patient and therefore more photons will reach the detectors, increasing the SNR.

14a. False **

An isotropic voxel is a cuboidal voxel that specifically is equal in length on all sides.

14b. True

This is true as long as the acquired voxels are isotropic and the axial images are contiguous.

14c. True

MPR is one of the most significant changes in CT in recent years. It allows reformatting of images to give true coronal and/or sagittal images even if the patient was rotated in the scanner, which can significantly aid in interpretation. It can also allow several layers to be added together to create thicker slices with a much better SNR, a technique often used in CT brain interpretation.

14d. True

3D images which can be rotated are useful in showing blood vessels adjacent to bony structures, while 3D surface rendering allows 3D fly-through techniques such as those used in virtual colonoscopy interpretation.

14e. False

MIP images show the maximum HU value for each column of voxels selected, and so are useful in following high intensity structures such as blood vessels with contrast. Minimum intensity projection (MinIP) can be used to follow the bronchial tree.

15a. False ***

This occurs when an extremely dense object (e.g. hip replacement) limits beam penetration and the very low signals received from the beam passing through that structure are outside the range that can be accurately processed.

15b. False

The opposite is true. Beam hardening removes the lower energy photons which may cause an error in the calculation of the HU of deeper voxels. The higher penetration of the deeper resulting beam leads to lower attenuation coefficients and HU to be measured. Lower HUs are displayed as darker pixels on the monitor.

15c. True

This is less apparent with multi-slice due to sampling overlap.

15d. True

If the object is smaller than a voxel its high density will be averaged across that whole voxel so it will seem bigger and less dense.

15e. False

Although objects at the centre of rotation are always represented by the same central detector(s), as the scan progresses these same objects will move out of the central plane and then be represented by the outer detectors thus contributing to the potential cone beam artefact. The cone beam effect will, however, be less at the rotation axis compared with objects at the scan periphery.

16a. False ***

A dark or light ring may be caused by a detector fault, but this is known as a ring artefact, although on spiral multi-slice CT it would be seen as a spiral with only a section of the circle being seen in a transaxial slice. Photon starvation describes an area that is poorly imaged and dark due to blocking of the beam photons by high attenuation objects such as hip prostheses.

16b. True

By creating a contiguous data-set and scanning volumes very quickly, there is less chance of slice misregistration.

16c. True

Although motion artefacts are reduced by faster CT scans, any movement within the time of the scan will result in motion artefact or blurring, especially in ill patients who may not be able to hold their breath or understand to keep their head still.

16d. False

Metal correction algorithms do exist, but can only partially compensate for the streak artefacts caused. Metal dental amalgam can significantly limit the information obtained during head and facial bone CT, and metal prostheses significantly limit the images of the pelvis.

16e. True

If the object is smaller than a voxel or only partially fills a voxel the HU of that voxel will be the average of the object and any other material within the volume that voxel represents. This may result in small lesions such as calcified granulomata being registered as soft tissue density. This is called the partial volume effect.

17a. False ***

In general terms this is true due to the extra half revolution required at either end of the scanned volume for interpolation when using multi-slice. Post-patient collimation and decreased geometrical efficiency in single-slice could potentially balance out this difference in dose.

17b. True

Assuming other scan parameters are unchanged, an increase in pitch will reduce dose by scanning through a larger patient volume in each rotation of the gantry. Pitch greater than one means there are gaps in the data-set.

17c. True

CTDI is a measure of the average dose at a specified location within the slice thickness.

17d. False

In general, dose is independent of slice thickness assuming the same volume is scanned and the same kV and mA are used.

17e. False

It is the mAs that are modulated as described.

18a. False ***

It is usually measured with a pencil ionization chamber to enable calculation of the dose from a single rotation of the gantry or per slice.

18b. True

This equates to approximately 4 years of normal UK background radiation.

18c. False

A CT KUB has an effective dose of 10–15 mSv. An X-ray IVU has an effective dose of 1.5–3 mSv.

18d. False

Multi-slice scanners do increase patient dose; the beam is collimated slightly more than required to ensure accuracy of image processing and there is also oversampling at the beginning and end of the volume acquisition to allow two-point interpolation. The increase in dose is in the region of 10%.

18e. False

The sum of the entry and exit doses for each projection is generally greater than the central dose such that the centre gets a lower dose than the periphery for a complete rotation. The difference gets less marked for smaller cross-sectional areas, for example in the head the dose is more uniform within the cross-section.

19a. True ***

This is accounted for by the much higher doses used in each CT examination compared with plain radiographs such as chest radiographs.

19b. False

The CTDI gives a measure of the dose from a single rotation of the gantry. $CTDI_{vol}$ gives the average absorbed dose within the volume of a defined width and is partially determined by the pitch.

19c. False

$DLP = CTDI_{vol} \times$ the length of the scanned area. It gives the absorbed dose of the scan. The DLP can then be adjusted by conversion coefficients based on the tissue weighting of affected organs to give an approximate effective dose.

19d. True

Roughly equivalent to an average yearly background radiation dose in the UK.

19e. True

Roughly equivalent to around 3 years of average background radiation dose in the UK.

20a. False **

Special sequences can allow 3D images at 5 frames per second or greater for biopsy needle placement. Other sequences can be set at a lower than normal dose for CT. Alternatively, biopsy needles can be placed and moved with scanning done at intervals while the operators briefly leave the room.

20b. True

Guidelines advise caution with an estimated glomerular filtration rate (eGFR) of 30–60. An eGFR of below 30 is associated with significant risk associated with iodinated contrast injection. Injection of contrast has to be balanced with the risk of nephrotoxicity and other risks compared with the extra information gained from a contrast study.

20c. False

A true anaphylactic reaction is fortunately a rare occurrence. Many hospitals have a policy that a doctor should be available to call in an emergency should this arise, however, as it can be potentially life threatening.

20d. True

Intramuscular adrenaline and airway management are the most urgent steps in treating an anaphylactic reaction. Further management may include corticosteroids, antihistamines and intravenous fluids. In a true anaphylactic reaction additional help from emergency medical or anaesthetic personnel should be sought rapidly. Thorough knowledge of local guidelines before such an event occurs is advised.

20e. True

Multi-slice detector scanners with 256 or more rows of detectors can scan the entire heart in less than one full rotation, which is fast enough to avoid motion artefact of the beating heart.

1. **Regarding radioactivity:**
   a. All stable nuclei have equal numbers of protons and neutrons
   b. Isotopes are nuclides of the same element which have differing numbers of neutrons
   c. Radionuclides are by definition unstable
   d. Most radioactive substances occur naturally
   e. The Systèm International (SI) unit of radioactivity is the becquerel (Bq)

2. **Concerning isotopes:**
   a. Radionuclides occur naturally and are present in the body at all times
   b. They will always have the same position in the periodic table
   c. The atomic mass number is the same for all isotopes of a given element
   d. Neutron deficit is defined as a nucleus with fewer neutrons than protons
   e. ^{99}Technetium (Tc-99) has a physical half-life of 6 hours

3. **Radioactive decay:**
   a. Can occur in nuclides with either a neutron excess or a neutron deficit
   b. In β^- decay, the mass of the nuclide is unchanged but the atomic number will have increased
   c. Isomeric transition means only the energy state of the nuclide changes
   d. A neutron deficit can be balanced by combining a K-shell electron with a proton to create an extra neutron
   e. Emitted gamma rays will vary in their energy from different atoms of the same radionuclide

4. **In radioactive decay of a nucleus the following result in a decrease in atomic mass number:**
   a. K-shell capture
   b. Positron emission
   c. Alpha particle emission
   d. Beta particle emission
   e. Isomeric transition

5. Regarding positrons:
a. A positron has an identical charge to a proton
b. A positron has an identical mass to a photon
c. Positrons are captured by the positron emission tomography (PET) scanner detector array to produce a three-dimensional (3D) map of nucleus decay
d. Positrons are an example of β emission
e. Positrons are likely to be emitted by a nucleus with a proton deficit

6. Regarding half-life:
a. Radioactive decay is a predictable process; it can be calculated when a given atom will undergo transformation
b. Decay occurs linearly
c. In clinical use of radionuclides, only the physical half-life is important
d. If the physical half-life is 6 hours and the biological half-life is 3 hours, in 6 hours the total activity of a radiopharmaceutical will have fallen by a factor of 8
e. In clinical use a half-life of several days is desirable

7. Concerning the decay of radionuclides:
a. When I-131 decays to Xe-131 a positive beta particle is released
b. Molybdenum-99 (Mo-99) decays by isomeric transition into ^{99}Technetium metastable (Tc-99m)
c. Positrons emitted by the decay of Flourine-18 (F-18) have energy of approximately 511 keV
d. It is possible for radiopharmaceuticals labelled with Tc-99m to have an effective half-life of over 24 hours
e. Activity of a radionuclide is described by the number of nuclei decaying per second

8. Radionuclides:
a. Are generally safe to be injected directly into the patient
b. Ideally emit alpha particles when used in a clinical setting
c. For medical use can be created locally in a cyclotron
d. That are isotopes of their parent nuclide are easily separated for clinical use
e. Are not radioactive until they are injected into the patient

9. Concerning the production of radionuclides:
a. Mo-99 is manufactured in a cyclotron
b. Creating a radionuclide with a neutron deficit does not change the atomic number
c. Radionuclides for use in medical imaging can be obtained from spent fuel rods from industrial nuclear reactors
d. F-18 has a half-life of 2 days
e. Tc-99m has a half-life of 200 000 years

10. **Radiopharmaceuticals:**
    a. The effective half-life is always shorter than the physical half-life
    b. The effective half-life is the product of the physical half-life and the biological half-life
    c. A diagnostic radiopharmaceutical should ideally emit monoenergetic gamma rays of 50–300 keV
    d. A diagnostic radiopharmaceutical should ideally not emit alpha or beta particles
    e. For intravenous radiopharmaceuticals, patients are normally advised to empty their bladders frequently

11. **Concerning radiopharmaceuticals:**
    a. The biological half-life of the pharmaceutical tagged with the radioisotope should never be longer than 60 min
    b. The generator for manufacturing Tc-99m has to be replaced once a month
    c. Tc-99m is used widely in radionuclide imaging because it can be tagged to a variety of compounds and is a pure beta emitter
    d. Patients often self-inject radiopharmaceuticals to reduce radiation dose to staff
    e. Only an Administration of Radioactive Substances Advisory Committee (ARSAC) certificate holder can handle and administer radiopharmaceuticals

12. **Tc-99m:**
    a. Has an atomic number of 99
    b. Is created from Mo-99 when it undergoes β^- decay
    c. Decays to its isomer Tc-99 with a half-life of 6 hours and the release of a 140 keV gamma ray
    d. Is stable once it has undergone isomeric transition
    e. May be used in both dimercaptosuccinic acid (DMSA) and mercaptoacetyl triglycine (MAG3) renal scanning

13. **Regarding the gamma camera used for planar imaging:**
    a. Simultaneously creates images of radioactive distribution in many planes
    b. They can only detect gamma radiation
    c. Sodium iodide (NaI) is sensitive to the gamma radiation of Tc-99m
    d. The position of an incident gamma photon in the camera crystal is determined by a few large photomultiplier tubes
    e. A photomultiplier transforms light photons into electrons which can be read as an electrical signal that represents light intensity

14. **Concerning the structure and function of a gamma camera:**
    a. The lead collimator contains septa that are 3 mm thick
    b. The detector array consists of multiple small NaI phosphor crystals coalesced into one
    c. Ideally patients should be situated a few metres from the crystal to reduce photon divergence
    d. Photomultipliers are used to increase the intensity of the light photon emitted by the crystal
    e. The use of a divergent hole collimator enables a larger field of view (FOV)

15. **The gamma camera:**
    a. The collimator is used to reduce scatter from the patient
    b. The NaI crystal is entirely covered in aluminium on all sides to prevent light entry
    c. A typical flash from a gamma photon would release in the order of 500 light photons
    d. The photomultiplier tube contains a series of dynodes at increasing positive potentials
    e. The pulse height analyser (PHA) rejects any signals that do not fall within set limits

16. **Concerning the pulse height analyser (PHA):**
    a. Scattered gamma rays will always be rejected by the PHA
    b. Pulse height is inversely proportional to the photon energy
    c. The sensitivity of the examination is increased by reducing the PHA window
    d. Multiple PHA windows may be used
    e. Pulses with energies of $\pm 30\%$ of the photo peak are normally allowed through

17. **Collimators, spatial resolution and sensitivity:**
    a. A collimator with more and smaller holes will increase sensitivity
    b. A collimator with more and smaller holes will improve spatial resolution
    c. A convergent hole collimator may be used for small organs and children
    d. The sensitivity of a typical collimator is only in the region of 20–30%
    e. It is not possible to have maximum sensitivity and maximum spatial resolution using the same collimator

18. **SPECT:**
    a. Is an acronym for single photon emission computed tomography
    b. Measures gamma rays released from the annihilation of positrons
    c. Employs a rotating gamma camera(s) to analyse emissions from the patient
    d. Multiple axial sections are created simultaneously from one gamma camera
    e. Uses a continuously rotating gamma camera which takes measurements in one-degree increments around the patient

19. **Regarding the gamma camera images:**
    a. Spatial resolution is increased by using a thinner crystal
    b. The spatial resolution of a gamma image is similar to that of a 10 mm slice CT scan
    c. Signal to noise ratio (SNR) is increased by using a high resolution collimator
    d. SPECT images typically have a spatial resolution of 15–20 mm
    e. Filtered back projection is used when reconstructing SPECT images

20. **Image quality in SPECT:**
    a. The smallest detail resolvable is around 20 mm
    b. Quality control will ensure that gamma camera count rate sensitivity does not vary by more than 20%
    c. Resolution is worse for organs at depth
    d. Patient movement is not a problem due to the speed of gamma rays in air
    e. Multiple camera heads can improve resolution

21. **Regarding PET:**
    a. It commonly uses fluorodeoxyglucose
    b. The radionuclide used decays by electron capture
    c. The gamma photons released will always be of the same energy regardless of the radionuclide used to produce them
    d. Anatomic detail is high
    e. Patient dose is increased with longer scan times

22. **PET:**
    a. In a PET–CT scan the low dose CT scan is performed simply to enable anatomical correlation with the PET image
    b. F-18 is an unstable nucleus with a neutron excess
    c. Bismuth germinate solid-state scintillation detectors are used because of their long decay time and high detection efficiency
    d. Two detectors on opposite sides of the detector ring must register a photon at the same time for the event to be recorded
    e. Scan acquisition time is approximately 30 min for a body PET–CT

23. **PET scanner design:**
    a. A ring of approximately 1000 NaI detectors surrounds the patient
    b. Each detector has only one 'line of response'; that is with the detector directly opposite
    c. Photons detected within 10^{-9} sec of each other are considered simultaneous
    d. Time of flight PET improves image contrast
    e. 3D acquisition improves sensitivity

24. **Image formation in PET:**
    a. Is possible with detectors covering a 180° arc over the patient
    b. The activity measured in each detector is plotted as a sine curve to create a composite sinogram for all the data in each slice
    c. Uses filtered back projection
    d. Due to the duality of data acquisition, PET image reconstruction does not need to take account of tissue attenuation
    e. Data acquired in two-dimensions (2D) cannot be used for 3D imaging

25. **Quality assurance in gamma imaging:**
    a. Spatial resolution may be tested using a line source or a sheet source with a bar test pattern
    b. An area of persistently high or low counts using flood field testing could indicate photomultiplier defect
    c. A linear defect in the image may represent a cracked NaI crystal
    d. Persistently high count readings on all camera orientations may indicate contamination of the camera
    e. Collimators can be tested separately to determine its point spread function and modulation transfer function (MTF)

26. **Dose:**
    a. The organ absorbed dose depends on several factors including activity administered, fraction taken up by the organ, half-life of the radiopharmaceutical, energy and type of radiation and the length of scan time
    b. Effective dose for a Tc-99m lung ventilation and perfusion scan is in the region of 1.5 mSv
    c. A bone scan using Tc-99m will incur an effective dose of approximately 5 mSv
    d. Effective dose for a thallium 2-methoxy isobutyl isonitrile (MIBI) heart scan is in the region of 18 mSv
    e. Effective dose for an F-18 fluorodeoxyglucose (FDG) brain scan is in the region of 1 mSv

27. **Dose in radionuclide imaging:**
    a. Most of the administered radiation will deposit its energy in the tissue/organ of interest
    b. Most of the gamma rays released within the patient are detected
    c. Scan time does not affect dose
    d. A target organ will receive a lower dose than a source organ
    e. Staff can reduce their dose by holding radionuclides at arm's length and delivering them promptly

28. **Regarding the safety and handling of radionuclides:**
    a. The activity of a radionuclide dose is measured using an ionization chamber which is situated between the patient and the gamma camera
    b. The current measured in the ionization chamber of a radionuclide calibrator is dependent on the vessel in which the radionuclide is housed
    c. Vials containing Tc-99m radiopharmaceuticals should be stored in Perspex pots
    d. All spillages should be reported to the Health and Safety Executive (HSE)
    e. Doubling your distance from a syringe containing a radiopharmaceutical will reduce the dose by 50%

29. **Safety, accidents and disposal:**
    a. Gloves should be worn when handling radiopharmaceuticals as they provide protection from the gamma rays
    b. Radioactive material should be handled for the minimum amount of time
    c. A radiopharmacy should be classified as a controlled area under Ionising Radiation Regulations (IRR99)
    d. Pregnant patients and patients who are breastfeeding should never receive radiopharmaceuticals
    e. Vomiting and incontinence are treated as radioactive spills

7. Radionuclide Imaging: Answers

1a. False **

This is mostly true for light nuclei, except hydrogen. Heavy stable nuclei have an excess of neutrons; for example, those with atomic numbers greater than that of calcium (Z = 20) have more neutrons than protons. Also, not all isotopes with equal numbers are stable; F-18 used in PET scanning has nine protons and nine neutrons.

1b. True

The element is characterized by the number of protons in the nucleus.

1c. True

They achieve stability through decay.

1d. False

Approximately 2700 are known, most of which are man-made.

1e. True

1 Bq = 1 disintegration per second.

2a. True ***

Potassium-40 is present within our food and thus our bodies, and contributes approximately 7% of our average background radiation.

2b. True

With the same atomic number they are nuclides of the same element; this infers they also share chemical properties.

2c. False

All isotopes of the same element have an equal atomic number. The atomic mass number defines different isotopes.

2d. False

A neutron deficit is where an isotope could move to a lower energy level by increasing the number of neutrons or decreasing the number of protons. This may occur in an atom with fewer neutrons than protons, but hydrogen would be an example of a stable element with fewer neutrons that is not in neutron deficit.

2e. False

Tc-99 has a half-life of 200 000 years. Tc-99m has a half-life of 6 hours.

3a. True ****

With a neutron excess, the nuclide will undergo β^- decay; with a neutron deficit, positron emission or electron capture can occur.

3b. True

An extra neutron in the nucleus has been transformed into a proton (increased atomic number) and a negatively charged β particle is emitted.

3c. True

Following β^- decay the nucleus may be in a higher energy state. If this is not released immediately, then the nucleus is said to be metastable and will de-energize at a later stage through the release of a gamma ray.

3d. True
This is known as electron capture and leads to the release of characteristic radiation as the hole in the K-shell is filled from one of the outer shells.

3e. False
Gamma rays have characteristic energy for a given radionuclide. Beta rays are emitted with a spectrum of energy up to Emax, which is characteristic for the radionuclide.

4a. False ****
K-shell capture is an example of neutron deficit decay where a proton captures an electron from the K-shell to convert into a neutron. $P + e^- = N$. The atomic number has decreased, but the atomic mass number has remained the same.

4b. False
Positron emission is an example of neutron deficit decay, where the proton emits a positron to give off its charge and convert to a neutron. $P = N + \beta^+$. The atomic number has decreased, but the atomic mass number has remained the same.

4c. True
An alpha particle is two protons and two neutrons. This reduces the atomic number of the atom by two and the atomic mass number by four.

4d. False
β^- emission is an example of proton deficit decay where a neutron emits its charge in the form of an electron. $N = P + e^-$. The atomic number has increased, but the atomic mass number has remained the same. Positron emission is another type of beta emission.

4e. False
Isomeric transition is the emission of a gamma ray from a metastable isomer, such as Tc-99m. As no particle is emitted, both the atomic number and atomic mass number remain the same.

5a. True ****
Both positrons and protons have identical positive charge.

5b. False
Positrons have very little mass compared to protons, being equal to electrons in mass. A photon can be considered to have no mass.

5c. False
A positron collides with and annihilates an electron, producing two gamma rays of 511 keV travelling in opposite directions. The PET scanner detects these gamma rays.

5d. True
Both positrons and electrons are beta particles, sometimes labelled as β^+ and β^- respectively.

5e. False
Positrons can be emitted when a proton converts to a neutron, a type of decay in a neutron deficit atom.

6a. False ***

Decay does occur predictably, but by the laws of chance, i.e. it is known how long a proportion of the atoms in a sample will take to decay but not in which individual atoms this will occur.

6b. False

It occurs exponentially; over a given time (half-life) half of the atoms in a sample will have transformed, over the same subsequent time period the sample will have again reduced by half, etc.

6c. False

The physical half-life (t_{phys}) only accounts for the decay of the radio-nuclide. When a radionuclide is attached to a pharmaceutical and injected into a patient, we must also consider how this compound is removed from the body (biological half-life, t_{biol}).

6d. False

Using the formula $1/t_{eff} = 1/t_{biol} + 1/t_{phys}$ we calculate the effective half-life (t_{eff}) to be 2 hours in this example. In 6 hours therefore the total activity will have reduced by 8 (2^3).

6e. False

Ideally the half-life should approximate the length of the test undertaken. If the radionuclide is active in the patient for a long time after sampling is completed then they have received an unnecessary dose.

7a. False ***

I-131 has a neutron excess and decays to Xe-131 by releasing a proton and a negative beta particle.

7b. False

Mo-99 decays to form Tc-99m, which is a metastable radioisotope that undergoes isomeric transition.

7c. False

The energy of positrons depends on the radionuclide. They are positive electrons which travel about 2 mm in tissue before colliding with a negative free electron. This results in the release of 2 photons at 180° trajectories, each with an energy of approximately 511 keV.

7d. False

The effective half-life cannot be greater than the physical half-life, which in the case of Tc-99m is 6 hours.

7e. True

This is the definition of the SI unit of radioactivity, the becquerel (Bq).

8a. False **

Radionuclides are attached to pharmaceuticals to create compounds called radiopharmaceuticals. Ideally these should localize in the tissue of interest, be eliminated from the body with a half-life similar to the length of the study, and have a low toxicity.

8b. False

Alpha particles have a very short range in tissue, meaning they would not escape the patient; this would make detection difficult and transfer a very high dose to the patient. Ideally a radiopharmaceutical would emit gamma rays.

8c. True

F-18 with a half-life of 110 min is produced this way.

8d. False

As they are isotopes they have the same chemical and metabolic properties; this makes separation of a pure radionuclide difficult.

8e. False

They should always be handled with care, e.g. lead shielded containers and syringes, prepared behind a lead screen.

9a. False **

Mo-99 is manufactured in a nuclear reactor by adding an extra neutron to the nucleus and creating a neutron excess. In a cyclotron, a proton is accelerated into a stable nucleus, forcing out a neutron and creating a neutron deficit.

9b. False

The atomic number increases by 1.

9c. True

Mo-99 can be collected in this manner.

9d. False

F-18 has a half-life of 110 min. It is used in PET scanning.

9e. False

Tc-99m is a metastable isotope with a half-life of 6 hours. It decays to Tc-99 which has a half-life of 200 000 years.

10a. True ***

The effective half-life is the result of both the physical decay of the isotope and the biological excretion of the radiopharmaceutical.

10b. False

The reciprocal of the effective half-life is equal to the reciprocal of the physical half-life plus the reciprocal of the biological half-life: $1/t_{eff} = 1/t_{phys} + 1/t_{biol}$.

10c. True

This energy level is high enough to leave the patient, but not so high that detection is difficult.

10d. True

Alpha and beta particles lack the penetration to leave the patient and have a high linear energy transfer and so are more biologically damaging to the patient for no diagnostic advantage. In particular, alpha emitters should always be avoided due to their very high relative biological effectiveness (RBE).

10e. True

This helps to reduce exposure to the bladder and surrounding tissues. Obviously in a study to show reflux into the kidneys where the bladder needs to be full this advice would not be given until after the scan.

11a. False **

The biological half-life depends on the rate of metabolism and excretion of the substance. There are no exact limits. It needs to be long enough to enable a suitable diagnostic investigation, but as short as possible to reduce patient dose.

11b. False

The parent compound of Tc-99m is Mo-99, which has a half-life of 67 hours. The activity therefore diminishes at a rate that requires the generator to be replaced once every week.

11c. False

Tc-99m is used widely because it can be tagged to a variety of compounds and because it is a pure gamma emitter.

11d. False

That would be bad practice! Lead-lined syringes are used to reduce dose to staff.

11e. False

An ARSAC certificate is required for individual doctors who are permitted to undertake radionuclide imaging studies. However, the ARSAC certificate holder may authorize other suitably qualified individuals to prepare and administer the radiopharmaceuticals on their behalf.

12a. False ***

This is the mass number. Its atomic number is 43.

12b. True

This occurs in a technetium generator with a half-life of 67 hours.

12c. True

These features make it very useful clinically.

12d. False

Tc-99 has a very long half-life (200 000 years) and is not therefore stable.

12e. True

It can also be used in imaging the brain, heart, lung ventilation, biliary tree, liver, bony skeleton, spleen, etc.

13a. False ***

Planar implies the image is captured in only one plane; compare this with tomography using radionuclides, e.g. in SPECT and PET.

13b. False

A gamma camera is merely a crystal of NaI which has luminescent properties; other forms of radiation will stimulate it, but the PHA limits their inclusion in the image if they are not of the expected energy.

13c. True

This makes it suitable for use in gamma cameras used clinically, but other scintillants could be used.

13d. False

There are around 100 photomultipliers; these determine the position and intensity of incident radiation.

13e. True

5–10 light photons create a single electron; this is amplified around a million times to create a pulse of electricity that can be measured. The magnitude of this pulse is proportional to the energy of the original gamma ray.

14a. False **

The septa are typically 0.3 mm thick. The half-value layer of lead for Tc-99m is 0.3 mm.

14b. False

There is one large NaI crystal, which is typically 9–12 mm thick.

14c. False

Patients should be as close as possible to the crystal to maximize the radiation detected.

14d. False

The light photon strikes a photocathode which causes the release of an electron. This electron is then amplified through a series of dynodes in a photomultiplier to produce a recordable voltage.

14e. True

It has the effect of minimizing the image allowing a smaller camera to be used.

15a. False **

The collimator acts to ensure that the majority of the photons that pass through are travelling parallel to the direction of the columns. This is the closest thing possible to a usable lens, and without the collimator the image would be considerably more blurred.

15b. False

The NaI crystal is normally covered by aluminium on all sides apart from the side of the photomultiplier tubes. If it was covered on all sides it would not be possible to detect the light emitted following detection of a gamma photon.

15c. False

Typically around 5000 light photons are released.

15d. True

A single electron is released from the photocathode for every 5–10 light photons. These electrons are then accelerated through a succession of dynodes to release increasing numbers of electrons, until the final pulse received at the anode is approximately 10^6 times greater than the initial pulse from the photocathode.

15e. True

The PHA rejects pulses outside the photo peak as they are more likely to come from scattered radiation that would reduce the contrast of the final image.

16a. False ***

If the scattered rays create a pulse which falls within the PHA window then they may be registered.

16b. False

The greater the photon energy striking the photocathode, the greater the pulse height produced from the photomultiplier.

16c. False

Increasing the PHA window will increase the sensitivity but reduce spatial resolution due to increased scatter in the image.

16d. True

This is required when more than one energy of gamma ray is emitted, e.g. In-111.

16e. False

The window is usually set to $\pm 10\%$.

17a. False ***

More and smaller holes will exclude more incoming gamma photons from the patient, and thus the sensitivity will decrease.

17b. True

More and smaller holes will limit the angle the gamma photons can travel through the collimator at, and thus improve the spatial resolution.

17c. True

This allows a larger detector to be used than the imaged organ, which essentially magnifies the image. Obviously this is only possible if the organ is smaller than the detector.

17d. False

Typical sensitivity of a collimator is less than 1%.

17e. True

A high sensitivity collimator uses larger holes to allow more photons through resulting in a poorer resolution, and vice versa.

18a. True **

Use of the word *single* differentiates SPECT from the other 3D modality using radionuclides, i.e. PET (where two coincident photon emissions are detected).

18b. False

This is the source of gamma photons detected in PET. SPECT measures gamma rays released from the decay of radioisotopes, i.e. the same ones detected in regular gamma imaging.

18c. True

Compare this with PET, which has a ring of stationary detectors.

18d. True

The width of the camera in the z-direction is divided into equal sections; each section represents an image slice.

18e. False

Due to the low numbers of photons involved in image formation, the gamma camera will remain stationary for up to 30 sec. Typically images are collected in $6°$ increments.

19a. True ****

This reduces the distance the photon travels before reaching the photomultiplier and therefore improves intrinsic resolution. The sensitivity is reduced, however, when using a thinner crystal.

19b. False

With a planar image, the typical spatial resolution is 5 mm. A CT scan image has considerably higher resolution, generally about 6 lp/cm but up to 20 lp/cm for smaller FOV. 6 lp/cm is equivalent to a pixel size of about 0.85 mm.

19c. False
Noise is the greatest limiting factor of gamma camera images. High resolution collimators improve spatial resolution but at the expense of sensitivity. The proportion of quantum noise increases and SNR is reduced.

19d. True
SPECT is predominantly used to evaluate organ function rather than fine anatomical detail.

19e. True
It is a key component of the reconstruction process.

20a. True ***
The low number of photons involved and the consequent problems with noise in the image necessitate a larger-sized picture element than might otherwise be possible; as always there is a balance between spatial resolution and noise.

20b. False
Gamma cameras are tested for uniformity using a flood field; this should produce a uniform response across the camera. Variations of up to 2% are accepted; this is true for stationary and rotating cameras.

20c. True
With further to travel in tissue, gamma photons from deep organs undergo more attenuation. With more scatter and fewer photons in each picture element there is lower resolution. An attempt is usually made to correct for this.

20d. False
Each gamma photon will effectively be detected instantaneously. The problem is that scans can take a long time to complete. Movement unsharpness will be affected by these lengthy scan times, but due to the intrinsically poor spatial resolution, is not likely to be apparent in the final image unless there were very significant patient movement during the scan.

20e. True
With up to three gamma cameras detecting simultaneously, the requisite number of orientations are obtained up to three times as fast. This can reduce the effect of patient movement, or increase count rate for the same scan time. Both will lead to improved resolution in the image.

21a. True ***
Also known as FDG. The fluorine nuclide F-18 is radioactive, with a half-life of only 110 min.

21b. False
F-18 decays by releasing a positron. Note that both of these transformations occur due to a neutron deficit in the atom.

21c. True
When a positron and electron annihilate, their combined mass is completely turned into energy ($E = mc^2$). The mass of positrons and electrons is constant, so therefore is the energy of the gamma released (0.511 MeV). The source of the positron has no bearing on this.

21d. False

Structures which have very little or no FDG uptake will not be seen in a PET scan; many normal tissues therefore are not clearly represented. This is why PET is often fused with CT.

21e. False

As for SPECT, PET scanning measures radiation *emission*. After the radionuclide is administered, the patient dose is entirely dependent on the half-life and clearance from the body. Neither of these factors is affected by the scan time.

22a. False **

The CT scan does allow for anatomical correlation but also enables attenuation corrections to be made on the PET images.

22b. False

F-18 has a neutron deficit. During decay, a proton converts to a neutron with the release of a positron (positive electron).

22c. False

Bismuth germinate is used because of its short decay time (300 nsec). This allows for very rapid measurements and very little 'dead time'.

22d. True

The annihilation photons travel at almost 180° to each other and will register on diametrically opposite detectors practically simultaneously.

22e. True

This is a typical time of acquisition.

23a. False **

Bismuth germinate is used as it has a higher intrinsic efficiency for the higher energy photons used in PET; compare this to NaI used in lower energy SPECT. Current scanners have up to 30 000 detectors.

23b. False

Each detector will have a 'line of response' with many opposing detectors. The area of the scan plane covered by these describes a fan shape. In addition, recent scanners allow lines of response to detectors in adjacent rings in the z-direction.

23c. True

This is determined somewhat by the speed of the scanner electronics.

23d. True

Modern scanners are able to very precisely measure the time of photon detection. Time of flight PET uses minor time differences in detection to provide further position information; along a given line of response, the two gamma photons from positron annihilation will only truly arrive simultaneously if they arose at exactly the midpoint of the line. If the event occurred closer to one detector, that detector will receive the photon marginally sooner. Knowing the distance between detectors and the speed of photons allows that distance to be calculated. With better positioning, there is less blur in the reconstructed image.

23e. True

3D acquisition refers to the inclusion of coincident data between adjacent detector rings as well as those occurring in the plane of a single ring of detectors. For a given dose administered to the patient more events will be detected compared to 2D acquisition.

24a. False ***

Use of co-incident data requires that the patient is completely surrounded by detectors. CT and SPECT can function with only 180° of data acquisition.

24b. False

The activity in each point source within the image plane (i.e. each x-, y-coordinate) can be represented as a sine curve. The data from all the point sources in that image plane create a sinogram − think of a rope composed of many sine curve fibres.

24c. True

Sinogram data are analysed this way.

24d. False

The combined distance travelled through tissue for the two photons in PET is the same whether they arise deep in the patient or more superficially, a result of travelling at 180° to one another. Unlike CT and SPECT there is no reduction in signal for deeper structures. A correction for whole body tissue attenuation does need to be made, however; this is achieved with a transmission scan.

24e. False

2D acquisition means data are collected in one plane only (slices). As with CT this can be used to form 3D images.

25a. True *

The line source gives information to produce a line spread function and thus an MTF. The Bar test pattern gives similar information to line pairs in conventional radiology.

25b. True

Slight changes in the amplification of photomultiplier tubes can lead to visible alteration of the image. This needs to be tested on a regular basis.

25c. True

This would indicate that the crystal would need to be replaced.

25d. True

Contamination of radionuclide onto the gamma camera or collimator will result in higher counts being measured on all camera orientations, and lead to a reduction in the contrast of the image.

25e. True

This is determined at different distances from the point source and can then be used to help calculate system resolution at different distances from a patient.

26a. False ***

Length of scan time does not alter dose, as at the end of the scan there is no way to effectively remove the radiopharmaceutical. All the other factors mentioned do influence organ dose.

26b. True

This is equivalent to around 6 months of natural background radiation.

26c. True

This is the dose for 600 MBq administered activity.

26d. True

This is one of the highest doses commonly encountered with radionuclide imaging.

26e. False

8 mSv would be a more typical effective dose for this examination.

27a. False ***

Typically, only 20% reaches the area of interest.

27b. False

Gamma is released in all directions; even in PET the detectors surround only a fraction of the patient, so much of the gamma radiation goes undetected. Other factors such as tissue attenuation, collimator exclusion and losses to dead time reduce this further.

27c. True

These are emission studies; dose is entirely dependent on the activity administered.

27d. True

The American Society of Nuclear Medicine has developed a method of calculating organ doses; radioisotope accumulates in the source organs, which then irradiate target organs.

27e. True

Time and distance are basic principles for radiation safety.

28a. False ***

Before the radionuclide is administered to the patient, it is placed inside an ionization chamber (radionuclide calibrator) which records the ionization current produced by the emitted gamma rays. The current is proportional to the activity of the sample and is recorded in the patient's case-notes.

28b. True

The vessel type needs to be entered into the calibration equation when calculating the activity of a sample from the current recorded in the ionization chamber. In practice this is done automatically by selecting the vial/syringe type from a preselected list of vessels with known physical characteristics.

28c. False

Lead pots are required. Beta particles are absorbed by Perspex, gamma rays are not.

28d. False

This is not the case.

28e. False

If you double the distance from a point source of radiation, the dose will reduce to 25%. This is the inverse square law.

29a. False **

Gloves should be worn to prevent contamination resulting in an area of skin continually being exposed to radiation over a long period of time.

29b. True

Handling radioactive material significantly increases the radiation exposure because of the inverse square law. The time of this exposure should be kept to a minimum to limit total exposure.

29c. True

With large radionuclide activities held in the department it could be possible for staff to receive inappropriate doses; safety measures are of course in place to prevent this.

29d. False

Pregnant patients should ideally be offered an alternative method of imaging, the scan delayed until after pregnancy or the scan cancelled if not essential, as collected radiopharmaceutical in the bladder is in close proximity to the uterus. The scan may still be performed if the benefits are deemed to outweigh the risks of exposure to the patient and child. Some radiopharmaceuticals may be excreted in breast milk; advice should be given on the safety of breastfeeding and the time before breastfeeding should be allowed again if the scan is deemed necessary. Some radiopharmaceuticals are either not excreted in the breast milk, or they decay to negligible activity in 12 hours or less; studies can be performed with only minimal disruption to mother and child.

29e. True

Bodily fluids such as urine and vomit will contain radioactive material and therefore need to be treated in the same way as a spill. The spill should be cleaned and contaminated material should be safely disposed of or stored until radioactivity levels have fallen to a safe level. The area should be monitored to ensure that activity is at a safe level afterwards.

8. Ultrasound: Questions

1. Regarding ultrasound:
a. Clinically the range, 3 to 15 MHz is commonly used
b. Sound waves move through tissue as a zone of compression followed by a zone of rarefaction
c. It travels through tissue at 154 ms^{-1}
d. It is at the lower energy end of the electromagnetic spectrum
e. 30 decibels (dB) is a common energy used clinically

2. Concerning diagnostic ultrasound:
a. Ultrasound is a high frequency form of electromagnetic radiation
b. The reflective properties at the interface between tissues are utilized in image acquisition
c. The velocity is proportional to the atomic number of the material through which it travels
d. Damage to tissues from ultrasound causes a stochastic risk of cancer
e. M-mode ultrasound is the term used for mobile ultrasound units which utilize a single multifunctional transducer

3. Ultrasound waves:
a. Constructive interference occurs when two waves meet exactly out of phase
b. Do not undergo attenuation
c. Require a medium to travel in
d. Intensity is proportional to the square of the amplitude
e. The lower the frequency, the more penetrating the beam

4. Ultrasound in tissue:
a. All tissues attenuate ultrasound equally
b. The behaviour of ultrasound when it encounters an obstacle depends on the size of that obstacle relative to the wavelength of the sound
c. Specular reflection enables the visualization of tissue boundaries
d. A large difference in acoustic impedance between tissues means more sound is reflected and less is transmitted at their boundary
e. Since the angle of incidence equals the angle of reflection, ultrasound needs to hit a surface at approximately 90° to be detected by the same probe

5. Concerning the interaction of ultrasound with tissues:
   a. The acoustic impedance of a material increases proportionally with its density
   b. 70% of an ultrasound beam will be reflected at a gas–soft tissue interface
   c. Full reflection of ultrasound occurs when the wave encounters a structure that is much smaller than the wavelength
   d. Utilizing the high attenuation of a full bladder may allow diagnostic imaging of the deep pelvic structures to be performed transabdominally
   e. The half-value layer (HVL) distance of a beam is inversely proportional to its frequency

6. Acoustic impedance (z) and reflection:
   a. By imaging internally, endoprobes have a better impedance match to tissue than traditional external probes
   b. The proportion of the ultrasound wave reflected at a soft tissue interface is $R = (Z_1 - Z_2)^2/(Z_1 + Z_2)^2$
   c. If a beam cannot be transmitted due to a large impedance mismatch it will predominantly be refracted instead
   d. Coupling gel is used to reduce the reflection of the beam between the probe and the skin
   e. A high impedance object such as a rib or stone will appear as a bright object with an enhanced shadow

7. Attenuation, penetration and time gain compensation (TGC):
   a. An ultrasound beam is attenuated linearly in soft tissue rather than exponentially as with X-rays
   b. Attenuation of the ultrasound beam can be measured in decibels
   c. The attenuation coefficient of the ultrasound beam in soft tissue is proportional to the frequency
   d. At 3.5 MHz, the power of the returning beam after travel through tissue 15 cm deep would be approximately 100 times less than the initial power of the beam
   e. TGC can be used to electronically amplify signals returning from deeper structures to give a useful image

8. The piezoelectric effect:
   a. Voltage applied is directly proportional to movement produced, while in converse the pressure applied is indirectly proportional to the output voltage
   b. The resonant frequency of a transducer depends on the piezoelectric material used
   c. Resonant frequency occurs through constructive interference of sound
   d. Above a certain temperature, a piezoelectric element will lose this ability
   e. Direct current (DC) is most commonly used to drive ultrasound transducers in the clinical setting

9. **In the production of ultrasound:**
   a. The piezoceramic elements are commonly made from lead zirconate titanate (PZT)
   b. At the natural frequency of a transducer, the wavelength produced is equal to the thickness of the piezoelectric element
   c. A prolonged applied voltage will have a longer ring down time than a short pulse of the same amplitude
   d. A backing block absorbs waves produced by the back face of the piezoelectric element
   e. Matching layers serve to reduce the difference in acoustic impedance between the transducer and the patient

10. **Probe design:**
    a. Piezoelectric elements are naturally electrically conducting
    b. Acoustic coupling is required in the design of an ultrasound probe
    c. Damping reduces pulse duration in pulsed mode
    d. Focusing is not possible with a single piezoelectric element
    e. The width of each piezoelectric element in a multi-element array is usually around one wavelength of the sound produced

11. **Concerning ultrasound transducers:**
    a. Ultrasound probes have no moving parts and are therefore not easily damaged if dropped
    b. The long wavelength beam produced by endoprobes (e.g. transvaginal) improves spatial resolution but reduces the depth of penetration
    c. PZT piezoceramics can function in temperatures up to about 500°C
    d. A high pulse repetition frequency (PRF) enables pulsed Doppler measurements of high velocity flow
    e. The 3rd harmonic of a 3 MHz transducer will be 300 MHz

12. **Multi-element ultrasound transducers:**
    a. An annular array is focused in two dimensions
    b. Electronic focusing creates a shorter focal distance if the delay between energizing individual elements is increased
    c. All of the piezoelectric elements contribute to the beam at all times in a stepped linear array
    d. A phased array can perform electronic sector scanning
    e. With several rows of elements, electronic focusing can also be applied across the plane of slice thickness in a linear array

13. **The ultrasound beam:**
    a. Maintains its dimensions indefinitely
    b. The near field is longer with a higher frequency
    c. There is less near field divergence with an increasing transducer diameter
    d. The bandwidth of useful frequencies in an ultrasound beam is wider for transducers with high damping
    e. Side lobes occur at the distal end of the primary beam

14. **Image formation in ultrasound:**
    a. A-mode scanning is utilized in most modern scanners
    b. Time gain compensation is not needed in B-mode scanning
    c. B-mode provides spatial information only
    d. During scanning, more time is spent receiving than transmitting echoes
    e. The difference between static and realtime B-mode imaging is that frames need to be reproduced more than 100 times per second in realtime

15. **With realtime ultrasound imaging, if all other factors are kept constant:**
    a. A higher PRF allows a higher number of lines per frame
    b. To view an object further from the probe the PRF must be increased
    c. The frame rate is inversely proportional to the PRF
    d. A typical abdominal ultrasound at 20 cm maximum depth might allow 100 lines per frame and 30 frames per second (fps)
    e. Frame rate × lines per frame = Velocity of sound in tissue/ depth × 2

16. **Contrast and harmonic imaging:**
    a. Contrast agents used in ultrasound include microbubbles or nanoparticles up to 1 mm diameter
    b. Contrast agents increase the signal returned by resonating at the fundamental and harmonic frequencies
    c. Contrast agents can increase the sensitivity of ultrasound detection of pathology such as liver lesions
    d. Harmonics are frequencies that are multiples of the fundamental frequency
    e. Harmonic imaging requires a transducer with very little damping

17. **Artefacts in ultrasound:**
    a. Fluid filled structures often cause acoustic enhancement
    b. Speckle represents the true consistency of a solid organ
    c. Reverberation artefact is caused by a resonation of a small bubble that causes a track throughout the scan
    d. Reflection artefact can cause objects to appear in a different location
    e. Acoustic shadowing is of no use in ultrasound as it blocks the path of the beam

18. **Image artefacts with ultrasound:**
    a. Speckle occurs because there is nothing for the sound waves to reflect back from
    b. Shadowing occurs behind objects with a high attenuation coefficient
    c. Sound that has been multiply reflected will be placed less deeply in the image than the original reflective surface depth
    d. Refraction is compensated for in ultrasound imaging
    e. Reverberation artefact can be lessened with harmonic imaging

19. **Image quality in ultrasound:**
    a. The attenuation of a 3 MHz beam in a given tissue is less than that of a 10 MHz beam
    b. Streak artefact can occur when imaging the liver through the ribs
    c. The scanner interpolates data received from the transducer to fill in gaps between scan lines
    d. Macrobubble contrast agents can enhance visualization of blood vessels and liver metastases
    e. To achieve a frame rate of 25 fps with 100 lines per frame would require a PRF of at least 2.5 MHz

20. **Doppler:**
    a. The Doppler effect is the change in sound wave amplitude caused by reflection from a moving surface
    b. The Doppler effect is at a maximum when imaging blood vessels perpendicular to the beam
    c. In pulsed colour, Doppler flow that is too fast may be incorrectly coloured due to aliasing
    d. Aliasing does not occur in continuous wave Doppler
    e. In duplex scanning, if the angle θ of the blood vessel can accurately be measured, blood flow velocities can be calculated

21. **Concerning Doppler ultrasound:**
    a. Beam side lobes are not relevant to Doppler imaging
    b. Doppler enables the rate and direction of flow to be determined
    c. Pressure in a stenosed blood vessel can be estimated using the Bernoulli formula
    d. Duplex typically combines a Doppler image with A-mode imaging
    e. Using the Doppler equation shows that the reflected frequency is proportional to the speed of a moving interface

22. **Clinical use of Doppler:**
    a. Range gating is used for depth localization
    b. Continuous wave Doppler can be performed with a single transmit/receive probe
    c. The spectral trace only provides information on direction and mean velocity of flow
    d. A colour mapped Doppler image provides more accurate velocity data than spectral imaging
    e. Power Doppler is more sensitive in identifying flow than colour Doppler

23. **Quality assurance in ultrasound:**
    a. Ultrasound probe resolution can be tested by scanning a frame of wires immersed in a liquid
    b. A faulty transducer element in a linear array probe is not noticeable in the image since there are over 100 other functioning elements
    c. The Doppler function may be calibrated using a Leeds test object
    d. Ultrasound can be tested using gelatine based phantoms
    e. Mechanical Index (MI) describes the manoeuvrability of the beam with a phased array

24. **Image quality in ultrasound:**
    a. Axial resolution is improved with lower frequency ultrasound
    b. Lateral resolution is best in the focal zone
    c. Phantoms for testing resolution consist of a solid Perspex box with a variety of copper rods of different diameters running through them
    d. Quality assurance requires that distance measurements are accurate to 0.2%
    e. Tissue mimicking phantoms can be used to assess greyscale

25. **Ultrasound resolution:**
    a. Axial (depth) resolution in ultrasound is better than lateral resolution
    b. Axial resolution is proportional to the wavelength of the sound
    c. Lateral resolution is the ability to distinguish two objects perpendicular to the direction of the wave
    d. The lateral resolution is approximately equal to the beam width at the depth of the objects
    e. Lateral resolution for ultrasound focused at 5 cm depth would be in the region of 1 mm

26. **Ultrasound safety:**
    a. Staff using ultrasound should be mindful of the Ionising Radiations Regulations 1999 (IRR99)
    b. Time averaged intensity should nowhere exceed 100 mW/cm^2 and total energy should not exceed 50 J/cm^2
    c. The intensity of the ultrasound beam at the focal region averaged over the course of the examination is approximately 10 mW/cm^2
    d. The power of an ultrasound probe may be measured with a force balance used to assess the sound pressure
    e. The Thermal Index (TI) is the ratio of the power output divided by the power required to raise the temperature of the tissue by 1°C

27. **Safety in ultrasound:**
    a. The British Medical Ultrasound Society (BMUS) produces safety guidelines for the use of diagnostic ultrasound
    b. It is bad practice to hold the probe stationary for extended periods of time while it is transmitting ultrasound
    c. Pulsed Doppler is used routinely in eye examination
    d. An MI > 0.7 indicates a potential risk of cavitation
    e. With a TI of 1.0, fetal scanning should be limited to 30 min

28. **Guidelines for the use of ultrasound:**
    a. MI should not be greater than 0.7 if a contrast medium is used
    b. MI > 0.3 should not be used in non-diagnostic fetal ultrasound scans
    c. MI > 0.3 should not be used in fetal ultrasound scans
    d. According to BMUS guidelines, the abdomen of a pyrexial adult patient (38°C) can safely be scanned for up to 45 min at a TI of 3
    e. Ionising Radiation (Medical Exposure) Regulations (IR(ME)R) state that justification of ultrasound requests must only be made by a registered medical practitioner

1a. True **
3 MHz might be used on an abdominal probe, 15 MHz for examining an eye.

1b. True
The total length of these two zones is equal to the wavelength of the sound.

1c. False
Ultrasound travels through tissue at approximately $1540 \, ms^{-1}$.

1d. False
Ultrasound is not a form of electromagnetic radiation.

1e. False
No universal reference intensity exists for ultrasound. Decibels are used to indicate a change in intensity from say, the transmitted energy. The decibel scale is logarithmic to the base 10 such that a doubling of intensity adds 3 dB, while increasing output by 10 times adds 10 dB.

2a. False ***
Ultrasound waves are longitudinal mechanical waves.

2b. True
This occurs due to differences in acoustic impedance.

2c. False
The velocity of the wave equals the wavelength × frequency. In tissue, the velocity depends on the density and compressibility of the tissue.

2d. False
To date no link between cancer and ultrasound exposure has been made.

2e. False
M-mode ultrasound is used to visualize rapidly moving structures (e.g. heart valves) which are displayed on the screen as a composite of A-mode images in an image which shows the motion (y-axis) versus time (x-axis).

3a. False **
This describes *destructive* interference where waves can cancel each other out; constructive interference occurs if waves meet exactly in phase. In this latter scenario their amplitudes are added.

3b. False
Although occurring by very different mechanisms to ionizing radiation, ultrasound waves also undergo absorption, scattering and reflection.

3c. True
Like all sound, ultrasound waves cannot travel through a vacuum.

3d. True
Knowing the intensity of the beam is important for issues of safety.

3e. True
Sound energy is absorbed as heat; this increases exponentially with depth and is greater for higher frequencies.

4a. False ***

Each tissue has its own ultrasonic attenuation coefficient. These are usually expressed as decibel loss per cm of tissue per MHz. Although they also vary within and between individuals, on average soft tissues attenuate 0.5 – 1.0 dB/cm. In muscle it can be 3 dB/cm, for bone 20 and in fat 0.6. Remember these are the single pass values; the effect is therefore doubled after sound has been both sent and received.

4b. True

If the object is larger than the wavelength, the beam will remain intact but may change direction/be reflected. With smaller objects, the beam's energy is scattered.

4c. True

This is the scenario when an object is larger than the wavelength of the sound.

4d. True

Acoustic impendence (z) is defined as $\sqrt{}$(bulk modulus $\times$ the density of the material). Bulk modulus (K) is a measure of compressibility. With a greater difference in z, more sound is reflected and less is transmitted. This is important clinically where the ultrasound beam meets the narrow air gap between the probe and the skin as there is naturally a large mismatch between the two; acoustic coupling is therefore required.

4e. False

In clinical use an angle of incidence of $90 \pm 3°$ is ideal. However most interfaces in the body also return scattered echoes and so can still be visualized at angles well away from $90°$.

5a. False ***

It increases proportionally with the square root of the density, i.e. Acoustic impedance $= \sqrt{}$(bulk modulus $\times$ density).

5b. False

Over 99% will be reflected.

5c. False

This causes scatter in all directions. Some of the scatter returns to the probe and contributes to the image, e.g. the signal obtained from tissue parenchyma.

5d. False

Water and urine have a very low attenuation. This allows the wave to pass through with very little absorption or scatter and may aid the ultrasound penetration.

5e. True

The penetration of the beam does reduce proportionally with frequency. Although not commonly described in these terms, ultrasound attenuation can be estimated in the same way you calculate HVL for X-rays; exponential decay and an attenuation coefficient proportional to frequency give a half-value distance that is inversely proportional to frequency.

6a. False ***

The technology in the probe is very similar and there is still a large native impedance mismatch between the piezoelectric element and soft tissue.

6b. True

Typical reflection proportions would be 99.9% air–tissue, 30% bone–muscle, 1% fat–muscle.

6c. False

A large impedance mismatch predominantly causes reflection of the beam. Refraction occurs when a beam is transmitted past an interface.

6d. False

Without coupling gel the beam would effectively be blocked by the interface of probe–air–tissue; it is therefore a requirement.

6e. False

A stone or rib will appear as a bright reflection with a dark *unenhanced* area of shadow, as no signal will be able to return from the area blocked by the object.

7a. False ****

The attenuation of the ultrasound beam in soft tissue is exponential.

7b. True

The decibel $= 10 \times \log_{10}$ (ratio of power). A change of 3 dB is approximately equal to a doubling or halving of the power.

7c. True

This explains why lower frequency probes are used for deep structures such as abdominal scanning despite the better resolution of higher frequency probes. Roughly penetration $= 40$/frequency.

7d. False

The returning beam would be about 100 dB less, which is 1/10 000 000 000.

7e. True

The signals from deeper structures are amplified electronically by a factor that increases the further away a structure is. This gives a useful picture where objects further away are presented with roughly the same brightness as closer objects despite returning a signal that may be many thousands of times weaker.

8a. False **

The effect is equal in both directions, i.e. input voltage is proportional to movement produced, while pressure applied is proportional to voltage out. This enables one piezoelectric element to be used in both the generation and detection of ultrasound.

8b. True

Resonant frequency is that at which a piezoelectric element would naturally reverberate at. Although it can function at any frequency, it is most efficient at its resonant frequency. This is determined by both the composition and the dimensions of the element; its width is equal to half the wavelength of the resonant frequency ultrasound.

8c. True

As the first sound wave leaves the face of the transducer, an equivalent wave travels backwards through the element. At the resonant frequency, this wave is reflected from the far edge and returns to the output face at exactly the same time as the next forward moving wave. Constructive interference therefore occurs since the waves are completely in phase.

8d. True

Known as the Curie temperature, for PZT it is around 350°C.

8e. False

B-mode scanning, the most common form used in clinical imaging, uses pulses of ultrasound; these are provided by short repetitive bursts of alternating current (AC).

9a. True ****

They can also be made from plastic polyvinylidine difluoride (PVDF).

9b. False

The natural or resonant frequency is that which produces a wavelength equal to twice the thickness of the element. This results in a maximum constructive interference between the forward travelling wave and the wave reflected from the back of the transducer.

9c. False

Mechanical damping from a backing block ± electronic damping from a briefly applied reversed voltage determines ring down time.

9d. True

It has similar acoustic impedance to the transducer.

9e. False

The acoustic impedance of the matching plate lies in between that of the transducer and patient. This allows a greater transmission of energy, but it does not reduce the difference in acoustic impedance between the ceramic transducer element and the body. In the same way, stairs do not reduce the difference in height between two floors in a building, they enable a smooth transition.

10a. False ***

An electrically conducting coat is applied to the piezoelectric element.

10b. False

Although ultrasound gel provides a necessary link between the probe and skin, acoustic coupling is also included in the probe itself. PZT and skin have a large impedance mismatch; only 20% of sound would naturally be transmitted. The probe membrane has an acoustic impedance intermediate between that of PZT and soft tissue thus reducing this mismatch and improving sound transmission.

10c. True

Akin to placing a hand on a ringing bell, damping limits resonance in the element following application of voltage. This is used to ensure short pulse duration in pulsed mode scanning.

10d. False

Focusing of a single element can be achieved with a curved element or by including an acoustic lens in the design. Modern probes achieve focusing with multiple elements (linear or annular) which are fired sequentially from the outermost in.

10e. True

Sound spreads out evenly in all directions from each element in a multi-element transducer when they are equal in width to one wavelength. Constructive interference between these multiple simultaneous waves creates a forward propagating beam. In a single element probe, the diameter is usually around 20 times the wavelength.

11a. False **

Dropping an ultrasound probe can cause cracks in the probe element and anger in your consultant. Heating may also damage the element, and thus probes are sterilized with alcohol wipes and not autoclaved.

11b. False

High frequency (low wavelength) beams give improved resolution but with reduced penetration.

11c. False

Above a certain temperature, materials lose their piezoelectric properties. This is the Curie temperature and for PZT it is approximately 350°C.

11d. True

This comes at the expense of range/depth of measurement.

11e. False

Harmonics are multiples of the original frequency. The 3rd harmonic is $3 \times 3 = 9\,\text{MHz}$.

12a. True ***

An annular array has multiple concentric rings of piezoelectric element. These focus to the point of a cone, i.e. in all planes perpendicular to the beam. A linear array by converse is only focused in one dimension; the other has to have separate focusing.

12b. True

Electronic focusing works by energizing the outermost pair of elements first then sequentially moving in after a short delay. Constructive interference leads to formation of a beam which has a focal length determined by the delay between neighbouring elements. With a greater delay the outer beams will travel further than the inner, thus flattening the triangle of focus and bringing the focal point closer.

12c. False

The elements are energized sequentially in overlapping groups of perhaps six at a time; usually there are 128 or 256 elements in total. This creates a series of parallel beams that are used to form an image line by line.

12d. True

By phasing the current from one end of the scanner to the other, the beam can be steered electronically. This can be adjusted between pulses to create a beam that sweeps from side to side and thus performs sector scanning.

12e. True

This improves image resolution.

13a. False ****

Constructive interference of adjacent sound waves arising perpendicularly from the face of an ultrasound probe leads to reinforcement and the creation of a beam. Parallel to this but beyond the edges of the transducer, destructive interference ensures this beam has a defined rectangular shape. This region is known as the near field or Fresnel zone. As sound moves further from the transducer, the dual effect of sound interference is lost and the beam begins to diverge; this is the far field or Fraunhofer zone.

13b. True

The length of the near field is proportional to: frequency $\times$ beam diameter^2.

13c. False

There is less far field divergence with a larger diameter transducer.

13d. True

Transducers with high damping can produce and respond to a greater range of frequencies; with more time to resonate a transducer will work towards its single, natural frequency.

13e. False

Side lobes are formed near the transducer due to small vibrations at the lateral edges of the piezoelectric element. These are comparatively of low intensity compared with the primary beam, but can cause artefacts.

14a. False ***

This stands for amplitude mode scanning and represents the simplest form of ultrasound imaging showing only the position of tissue planes. Modern two-dimensional (2D) imaging uses B(brightness)-mode scanning.

14b. False

Time gain compensation corrects for sound attenuation with depth. This is required in both A- and B-mode scanning.

14c. False

The brightness of each dot in the image directly relates to the amplitude of the signal received from that spatial location.

14d. True

Even with a PRF of 1 kHz (1000 pulses per second), only around 0.1% of the time is spent transmitting.

14e. False

Realtime imaging requires that B-mode frames are reproduced at least 25 times per second; this is sufficient for the human eye to perceive changes as movement. Scanners do sometimes drop to frame rates of 10–15 per second, but interpolate between frames so as to boost the refresh rate of the display and appear 'realtime'.

15a. True ***

PRF = lines per frame × frame rate.

15b. False

The further the object is from the probe, the greater the time for an echo to return, and therefore the PRF needs to be lower.

15c. False

The frame rate is proportional to the PRF.

15d. True

Scanning closer to the surface would allow higher frame rates and lines per frame.

15e. True

The depth is ×2 as the sound has to travel to the maximum depth and back again.

16a. False ***

Microbubbles are normally less than 4 μm and nanoparticles less than 1 μm. Both are used as contrast agents in ultrasound.

16b. True

Although the contrast agents are far too small to be resolved by the ultrasound beam, they resonate at the fundamental frequency and harmonic frequencies and generate a signal much larger than that from surrounding tissue and blood.

16c. True

Contrast agents taken up by vascular lesions can enhance lesions that would not otherwise be detectable on ultrasound imaging. They can also adhere to tissue walls and thrombus. Specialist contrast agents include immunologically-targeted microtubules.

16d. True

The distortion of the main frequency by its travel through tissue produces harmonics at multiples of the fundamental frequency. Although these echoes are at greatly reduced amplitude there are other advantages such as reduced scatter that make them useful for imaging.

16e. False

Harmonic imaging requires broad bandwidth transducers, which are normally heavily damped.

17a. True ***

Homogenous fluid such as urine in the bladder is weakly attenuating, and thus allows the beam to pass through and a better signal to be received from objects on the far side. This produces a bright area on the far side of the fluid structure. This effect is used in transabdominal gynaecological ultrasound, where the patient is asked to come with a full bladder to image the uterus and ovaries.

17b. False

Speckle does provide a textured appearance that can be interpreted, such as the bright appearance of a fatty liver. However, it is an artefact arising from the scatter of waves from structures that are too small to be resolved.

17c. False

Reverberation is where a wave is reflected several times within a structure close to the probe before returning and gives the appearance of a second object further away from the original. Reverberation within the probe and the gel is often seen as several bright lines across the field of view (FOV) at the top of the picture, and can sometimes mask objects very close to the surface. Resonation of a small group of bubbles describes the artefact of ring down.

17d. True

This can sometimes occur with objects within the liver reflecting off the smooth surface of the diaphragm and appearing to lie within the lung.

17e. False

Acoustic shadow can aid detection of gallstones and renal calculi and help to distinguish between calculi and polyps.

18a. False ***

Speckle occurs because the constituents of solid organ parenchyma are too small to fully reflect the sound. Instead, the beam energy is randomly scattered in all directions; some of this is detected, giving the characteristic speckled appearance of liver and spleen, etc.

18b. True

TGC will therefore under-compensate, making distal objects seem less echogenic. The opposite situation leads to acoustic enhancement.

18c. False

Multiply reflected sound will be placed deeper in the image than its true original reflective origin since the scanner assumes the sound has travelled in a straight line. The extra reflection(s) will delay its return.

18d. False

When sound is transmitted across a tissue boundary it will undergo some refraction. The ratio of the sine of incident and refracted angles is equal to the ratio of velocity in the two tissues; this is Snell's law. Ultrasound scanners assume travel in straight lines, there is no compensation for refraction.

18e. True

This occurs when multiple reflections occur between the transducer and an interface near the surface, creating lines parallel to this interface.

19a. True ****
The attenuation (decibel loss per centimetre) of a beam is proportional to the frequency.

19b. False
This could cause acoustic shadowing, where a high attenuation structure reduces the intensity of echoes received from deeper tissues. Streak artefact is found in CT.

19c. True
This is especially needed at depth with a sector scanner since the scan lines are divergent.

19d. False
Microbubbles typically less than 4 μm in diameter are used as contrast agents.

19e. False
PRF = frame rate × lines per frame (2.5 kHz).

20a. False **
The Doppler effect is the change in frequency caused by reflection from a moving surface. The reflection of a wave from an object moving towards the wave effectively shortens the wavelength and increases the frequency. Reflection from an object moving away has the opposite effect.

20b. False
The Doppler shift is proportional to cos θ. At 90° (perpendicular to the beam) the Doppler shift will be zero. This can be seen when colour imaging a blood vessel where part of the vessel is coloured red, indicating flow towards the probe, the central part is black, showing no movement towards or away from the probe as the blood is flowing perpendicular to the beam, then a blue section indicates blood flowing away from the probe again.

20c. True
As the PRF is set by the maximum depth scanned, inadequate sampling may lead to aliasing errors, with fast flow being recorded as slow and vice versa.

20d. True
Continuous wave Doppler does not use pulses and therefore the sampling rate is not limited by the pulse repetition.

20e. True
This is clinically useful in many areas such as assessment of vessel stenosis.

21a. False ****
As with conventional imaging, they can cause artefacts. In Doppler it is possible to see a false signal.

21b. False
The rate of flow towards or away from the probe can be determined; direction of flow requires additional information from the B-scan image, i.e. the direction of any relevant blood vessel. This is duplex scanning.

21c. True

Flow velocity (v) increases through a stenosis. The pressure increases by 4 V^2. This is the Bernoulli formula. It gives an approximate value because it ignores the effects of blood turbulence and viscosity.

21d. False

Duplex scanning typically combines Doppler with B-mode imaging.

21e. False

It is the change in reflected frequency that is proportional to the speed of the interface.

22a. True ***

If detected, Doppler shift could be occurring anywhere along the line of the ultrasound beam. Range gating means the detector will only accept signal in a short window of time; since speed is constant, the time chosen is known to relate to a specific depth.

22b. False

Continuous wave Doppler requires two similarly aligned probes: one to transmit, one to receive.

22c. False

The spectral trace is a complete graphical representation of Doppler frequency against time. The Doppler signal is continuously sampled and each sample shows flow direction, component frequencies (equivalent to component speeds) and the number of blood cells at each frequency. From this the minimum, maximum and mean velocities can be calculated.

22d. False

Compared with spectral imaging, colour mapping is very limited. To produce realtime images with Doppler information, there is simply not enough time to sample more than 10 Doppler pulses per scan line. Thus, colour Doppler only provides information on direction, mean velocity and variance.

22e. True

Power Doppler only provides information on the amplitude of the Doppler signal; this depends on the number of elements involved in the flow irregardless of direction. Power Doppler is therefore more sensitive to identifying areas of low flow.

23a. True ***

The wires are spaced at decreasing intervals to test maximum resolution and are immersed in a liquid in which the speed of sound is 1540 ms^{-1}.

23b. False

The multiple elements in a linear array probe are not used simultaneously when imaging. Smaller groups are usually energized sequentially to provide a scanning beam; the effect of this means a single faulty element is more noticeable, usually as a dark streak on the image running parallel with the beam.

23c. False

The Leeds test object is commonly used in fluoroscopy quality assurance. Complex tissue mimicking phantoms can be used to test Doppler in ultrasound.

23d. True

These are used to check the accuracy of the greyscale picture in realtime imaging. Gelatine phantoms are created to closely represent tissue characteristics when examined with ultrasound.

23e. False

The MI measures the maximum amplitude of the pressure pulse in ultrasound; this is defined as the peak rarefaction pressure/frequency^2.

24a. False ****

Axial or depth resolution is the ability to differentiate two tissue planes in the line of the ultrasound beam; it is approximately half the pulse length. Pulses are shorter at higher frequency.

24b. False

Lateral resolution is the ability to differentiate two structures lying side by side at the same depth. This requires the beam to be narrower than the gap between the structures. A beam is narrowest in the focal zone.

24c. False

For assessing resolution, the phantom should be filled with fluid through which sound travels at approximately 1540 ms^{-1}. Solid Perspex is used to assess sensitivity and distance measures; these need to take account of the faster speed of sound in Perspex.

24d. False

2% is acceptable over a distance of 10 cm.

24e. True

These phantoms are made to represent solid organ parenchyma; the textural pattern created is assessed.

25a. True ****

Axial resolution is approximately three times better than lateral resolution.

25b. False

A higher frequency of wave and shorter duration of pulse results in a better axial resolution; this corresponds to a shorter wavelength, i.e. is inversely proportional.

25c. True

Axial resolution is the ability to distinguish two objects parallel to the direction of the wave.

25d. True

At the focal depth, beam width = focal length × wavelength/diameter.

25e. True

Improvements continue to be made to reduce the diameter of transmitting crystal needed and thus improve the resolution.

26a. False ***
Ultrasound does not use ionizing radiation, and thus does not fall under IRR99.

26b. True
Although these are agreed safety guidelines, there is no legal requirement to follow them.

26c. True
At an intensity of 10 mW/cm^2 it would take approximately 1 hour 20 min of imaging a single region to reach a total energy of 50 J/cm^2.

26d. True
This may also be done by measuring the heating effect with a calorimeter.

26e. True
The heating effect of an ultrasound probe may be used therapeutically, but can be of especial concern in antenatal scanning and in patients with a high fever. Guidelines exist on maximum scan length times depending on TI and patient core temperature.

27a. True ****
These are published online at www.bmus.org.uk

27b. True
This increases the energy transferred to a small volume of tissue, raising the possibility of thermal or mechanical damage. Care should especially be taken when using pulsed Doppler.

27c. False
The eyes, an embryo of less than 8 weeks gestation, and the central nervous system of a fetus or neonate are identified by BMUS as particularly sensitive targets for ultrasound examination; potentially high energy modes such as pulsed Doppler should therefore be avoided.

27d. True
This is a theoretical risk but 0.7 is the figure published by BMUS.

27e. True
Measurements of scanner outputs have shown that values of TI displayed on the screen can be too small. A TI of 1 may equate to a temperature rise of up to 2°C.

28a. True ****
There is a risk of cavitation if using contrast media. A theoretical risk of spontaneous cavitation also exists at an MI > 0.7 (BMUS guidelines note this as a threshold, and recommend that MI is kept to a minimum).

28b. True
A possible risk of minor damage to neonatal lung or intestine is reported at this level. BMUS guidelines recommend an MI < 0.3 for non-diagnostic scans.

28c. True
A possible risk of minor damage to neonatal lung or intestine is reported at this level.

28d. False

TI gives an indication as to the temperature rise in tissues as a result of the ultrasound beam. With a pyrexial patient, 10 min of scanning can be safely performed when TI = 2.

28e. False

IR(ME)R relates only to examinations using ionizing radiation.

9. Magnetic Resonance Imaging: Questions

1. **Regarding nuclear magnetic resonance (MR):**
   a. Only atoms with an odd number of either protons or neutrons exhibit magnetic resonance
   b. In a 1 T magnetic field a hydrogen atom proton will precess with a frequency of 42.6 MHz
   c. Placed in a powerful static magnetic field, all of the hydrogen atom protons in a patient will align themselves with this field
   d. The bulk magnetization of one million hydrogen nuclei in a patient will depend on a difference in alignment of only one nucleus in a 1 T magnet
   e. It is the combined magnetic vector of the hydrogen nuclei in a static field which provides the signal for MR

2. **Protons and magnetism:**
   a. Most medical magnetic resonance imaging (MRI) detects signals produced by the single protons of hydrogen nuclei
   b. Other nuclei with uneven numbers of protons or neutrons such as F-19 may also be used in MRI
   c. When placed in a 1 T field and before excitation, 'spin down' protons predominate
   d. Prior to any radiofrequency (RF) pulse the total magnetic vector in the xy plane (m_{xy}) is equal to 1
   e. A standard 1 T MRI scanner produces a field strength 100 times that of the earth's

3. **Regarding the MR signal:**
   a. The net magnetic vector in the z-axis provides a recordable MR signal
   b. The signal recorded in a 1.5 T magnet will be proportionally higher than in a 3.0 T magnet
   c. MR signal strength is inversely proportional to proton density
   d. RF transmitter/receiver coils need to be able to perform both functions simultaneously
   e. Most signals from the body are received from water protons

4. **The MR signal:**
   a. In the plane running transverse to the static magnetic field, there is no MR signal at rest
   b. Application of RF energy causes the hydrogen protons to precess in phase
   c. A 90° pulse requires more energy than a 180° pulse
   d. Following an RF pulse, the phase coherent protons will remain in this state indefinitely
   e. Depends only on the proton density of the material

5. **Signal formation:**
   a. The Larmor frequency is the frequency of precession of the protons
   b. Photons with twice the Larmor frequency have the correct energy to tip all the 'spin up' protons to 'spin down'
   c. Photons in a 180° RF pulse have twice the energy of photons for a 90° RF pulse
   d. An initial 90° RF pulse reduces m_z (the net magnetic vector in the z-axis) to approximately 0
   e. As the magnetic vector returns to its equilibrium position along z, a signal is produced which is received by an RF coil to form the picture

6. **Concerning T1:**
   a. It is the time taken for transverse recovery to reach 37% of the maximum value
   b. T1 is increased with greater field strength
   c. Fat and melanin both produce a high signal on a T1-weighted image
   d. A short time to echo (TE) and short time to repeat (TR) will give a T1-weighted image
   e. T1 is always longer than T2

7. **Concerning T2:**
   a. T2 decay is longitudinal relaxation
   b. A long TR and long TE will give a T2-weighted image
   c. Cerebrospinal fluid (CSF) and flowing blood will produce high signal on a T2-weighted image
   d. The T2 of grey matter is longer than that of white matter
   e. Spin–spin relaxation occurs because the neighbouring protons exert a tiny magnetic field of their own which can alter the rate of precession

8. **T2 decay:**
   a. Occurs due to spin–lattice relaxation
   b. Is referred to as T2* when an initial 180° pulse is used in spin-echo (SE) sequencing
   c. T2 relaxation time increases with an increase in magnet strength
   d. Is affected by magnetic field inhomogeneities
   e. When 63% of the transverse signal is lost, this is referred to as time T2

9. **T1 and T2 recovery:**
   a. Free induction decay (FID) is also known as spin–lattice relaxation
   b. T2 always has a longer decay time than T2*
   c. T1 time is the time for 63% recovery of m_z
   d. Fat and large molecules shorten the T1 time of tissues
   e. Local field variation is fastest in free fluids such as water, giving a short T2

10. **Basic MR sequencing:**
    a. FID is a commonly used basic sequence
    b. A spin-echo sequence removes the dephasing effect of field inhomogeneities with a second 90° pulse
    c. The rephasing pulse in SE sequencing also removes the need for ultrafast switching of coils from transmit to receive
    d. With improvements in magnet technology, field inhomogeneities will probably become a thing of the past, negating the need for the formation of spin-echoes in MR
    e. The longer the TE, the smaller the subsequent MR signal

11. **Regarding the SE sequence:**
    a. The SE sequence allows the T2 effect of a specific tissue to be measured
    b. The presence of the patient adversely affects the magnetic field
    c. Following rephasing, the MR signal is equal to that immediately after the initial 90° pulse
    d. Immediately following a single 90° pulse, all of the dipoles are in phase
    e. The 180° rephasing pulse is applied at TE/2 after the initial RF excitation

12. **Weighted images:**
    a. A T1-weighted image would have a TR of 1000 ms and a TE of 100 ms
    b. A T2-weighted image might have a TR of 400 ms and a TE of 15 ms
    c. Water and fluids such as CSF appear bright on T2
    d. Cortical bone appears white on proton density weighted images
    e. Short tau inversion recovery (STIR) is a type of fat suppression

13. **Imaging with MR:**
    a. Signal strength depends only on the proton density of the material
    b. A short TE and a long TR will give a T1-weighted image
    c. A T1-weighted image will show water as high signal
    d. Most soft tissues show as high signal on proton density (PD) weighted images
    e. If TE is longer than TR, the image is weighted towards PD

14. **Spatial encoding in MR:**
    a. Slice selection must always be applied to the z-axis
    b. In a standard SE sequence, frequency encoding is applied during signal acquisition
    c. In a standard SE sequence all of the information for a single slice is obtained within one TR
    d. The steeper the slice selection gradient, the thinner the slice
    e. In a standard SE sequence the image can be built up line by line during acquisition

15. Concerning spatial localization of the MRI signal:
    a. Slice selection is applied simultaneously with the initial RF excitation
    b. A row of phase encoding data in K-space takes less time to acquire than a column of frequency encoding data
    c. The centre of a K-space contains the data relating to high spatial resolution
    d. Slice thickness can be reduced by decreasing the RF bandwidth for each slice (assuming the gradient remains the same)
    e. RF excitation outside the field of view (FOV) can result in aliasing artefacts

16. Pulse sequences in MR:
    a. Within a single TR, following collection of PD-weighted data the echo can be re-sampled after another TE to provide T2-weighted data
    b. Inversion recovery is used to accentuate subtle differences in T1 weighting between tissues
    c. STIR sequencing is used to enhance tissue boundaries
    d. Gradient echo sequences achieve equivalent rephasing when compared to the 180° pulse of SE
    e. Echo-planar imaging (EPI) provides highly detailed images

17. Regarding imaging techniques and pulse sequences:
    a. Gradient recalled echo (GRE) sequences are used for their speed of acquisition
    b. Fast SE involves simultaneously recording multiple frequency encoding echoes which results in the acquisition time being shortened by a factor of 16 or more
    c. STIR sequences are used to suppress the signal from fat
    d. Multi-slice imaging is not possible in MR
    e. In diffusion-weighted images, tissue oedema produces a high signal

18. Other sequences and techniques:
    a. A reduced tip angle can be used to decrease the scan time at the expense of signal strength
    b. Fast (turbo) spin-echo (FSE) techniques use several refocusing 180° RF pulses to rephase and produce extra echoes at different phase gradients for each excitation
    c. Multi-slice MR techniques use several rows of detectors within the path of the beam
    d. In MR angiography flowing blood normally appears dark
    e. Gadolinium produces a bright area of uptake on T2-weighted images

19. **Advanced MRI:**
    a. Most MR contrast agents are paramagnetic
    b. In time of flight MR angiography, flowing blood shows as high signal because its movement prevents longitudinal relaxation
    c. Restricted diffusion shows as high signal and is abnormal in diffusion-weighted images of stroke
    d. Deoxygenated haemoglobin is paramagnetic; this is the basis for functional MRI
    e. Chemical shift imaging utilizes the subtle Larmor frequency differences for hydrogen contained in molecules to distinguish those molecules

20. **Concerning MR angiography:**
    a. On a SE sequence, slow flowing blood appears dark (flow void)
    b. In GRE flowing blood appears bright only after administration of intravenous gadolinium
    c. Pulsatile movement artefact is most apparent in the phase-encoding direction
    d. Vessel calcification will produce a high signal which can mask a stenosis
    e. Turbulent flow shows high signal on an SE sequence

21. **Artefacts in MRI:**
    a. Patient movement creates artefacts most commonly in the frequency encoded direction
    b. Flowing blood can appear bright in GE sequences
    c. Ferromagnetic foreign bodies appear as a high signal artefact
    d. Chemical shift artefact can be reduced through use of a steeper frequency encoding gradient
    e. Image wrap-around occurs only when using a magnet of less than 2 T

22. **Regarding MRI artefacts:**
    a. Chemical shift is displaced in the frequency encoding direction
    b. Chemical shift is more apparent at lower static field strengths
    c. Ferrous metal implants cause streak artefact
    d. Cardiac motion artefact can be reduced by triggering the pulse sequence with the electrocardiogram (ECG)
    e. Aliasing occurs if the FOV is too large

23. **Artefacts in MR:**
   a. Chemical shift artefacts are due to chemical diffusion and thermal movement in free fluid and oedema
   b. Chemical shift artefacts are in the phase encoding direction
   c. Aliasing may be apparent in the phase encoding direction as part of the image being wrapped to the wrong side
   d. Motion artefact occurs because the phase encoding steps are spread over time and therefore any movement can cause a misregistration of position
   e. Ferrous metallic objects can cause localized distortion and degradation of the image

24. **Image quality in MR:**
   a. Spatial resolution is better with smaller coils
   b. Surface coils improve signal to noise ratio (SNR) of near surface tissues
   c. SNR decreases as voxel volume increases
   d. T2 imaging always provides the best degree of tissue contrast
   e. For quality assurance purposes, magnetic field homogeneity should be tested daily

25. **Concerning MRI image quality:**
   a. Spatial resolution is reduced when using a thinner slice
   b. The majority of noise in an MR image is due to external RF interference
   c. Gadolinium nuclei emit the high signal seen on contrast-enhanced MR images
   d. Signal strength is increased by using a greater static field
   e. Some clinical sequences use simultaneous T1 and T2 weighting

26. **Image quality and noise:**
   a. Noise in MR is predominantly due to quantum mottle
   b. Noise is most apparent in areas of high signal such as fluid filled areas on T2
   c. Decreasing the voxel size improves the SNR and resolution at the expense of scan time
   d. Increasing TR and/or decreasing TE would increase the signal
   e. Increasing the number of excitations (N_{ex}) would increase the SNR at the expense of scan time

27. **Magnetic equipment in MRI:**
   a. The main system magnet must be a superconducting electromagnet
   b. Superconductivity requires cooling to near $0°C$
   c. Resistive electromagnets should ideally not be switched off
   d. Gradients for spatial encoding are provided by altering the main magnet
   e. The main magnetic field is normally defined to be along the z-direction

28. **Regarding the structure of a superconducting magnet MRI scanner:**
    a. A very large current is drawn from the electrical mains supply to maintain superconductance
    b. Quenching of the system may occur spontaneously if the operating temperature is not maintained
    c. A Faraday cage minimizes the effect of the scanner magnetic field beyond the boundary of the scanner room
    d. The field strength at 2 m from the centre of the magnet is 25% of the strength at 1 m from the centre of the magnet
    e. The use of surface coils gives greater image uniformity than body coils

29. **Different types of magnets and coils:**
    a. A 0.5 T superconducting magnet produces a greater field strength than a 0.5 T resistive magnet
    b. A paramagnetic MR system uses a conductive magnet
    c. A permanent magnet may be rapidly shut down in an emergency
    d. Shim coils are coils that are fine tuned to make the main magnetic field as uniform as possible
    e. Surface coils are placed directly on the patient

30. **RF coils in MRI:**
    a. Separate send and receive coils are needed
    b. The loud bangs heard during imaging occur when switching from transmit to receive
    c. Surface coils are commonly used for whole body imaging
    d. Phased array coils can allow faster imaging
    e. RF signal is amplified before transmission

31. **Equipment safety in MRI:**
    a. The torque effect is greater for rod-shaped objects
    b. Noise levels commonly exceed 90 dB
    c. The fringe field is well contained around an electromagnet
    d. Induced heating is the primary concern when using gradient fields
    e. A magnet quench can cause oxygen levels to drop in the scan room

32. **Concerning safety and MRI:**
    a. The Medicines and Healthcare products Regulatory Agency (MHRA) publishes guidelines on safe MRI practice
    b. A patient with a cardiac pacemaker should not be in an area where stray fields may be greater than 5 mT
    c. Ethics approval is not required for medical research scans under 2 T
    d. The presence of metallic dentition is a contraindication to MRI scanning
    e. Previous allergic reaction to iodinated intravenous contrast agents is a relative contraindication to administering gadolinium

33. **Safety issues:**
    a. Modern plastic cardiac pacemakers are safe for MRI
    b. Metal objects within the patient such as joint prostheses and past eye injury foreign bodies are not a risk to the patient as they are firmly fixed in place
    c. Patient screening should be performed as soon as the patient enters the controlled area
    d. Pregnant patients should not be exposed to field strengths above 2.5 T
    e. Specific absorption ratio (SAR) is the amount of ionizing radiation absorbed per mass of tissue expressed as watts per kg during the MR scan

34. **Safety in MRI:**
    a. Public access to areas where field strength is greater than 0.5 mT is restricted
    b. A patient with a pacemaker can have parts of their body other than the thorax imaged safely
    c. Routine whole body clinical scanning is limited to 4 T
    d. Torque force on joint replacements is of particular concern
    e. Varying gradient fields can cause nerve stimulation

35. **Regarding the effects of MRI scanning:**
    a. RF fields can cause peripheral nerve stimulation
    b. Equipment leads exposed to the gradient field can cause skin burns if inappropriately positioned
    c. Intraorbital metal fragments are of concern primarily because they can become overheated and cause thermal damage to the retina
    d. Staff with body piercings must wear lead-lined undergarments when approaching the magnet
    e. With a SAR of 1.0, the patient's body temperature will rise by more than 0.5°C if they are scanned for 30 min

36. **Emergencies in MR:**
    a. In the event of a cardiopulmonary arrest, the resuscitation team should never enter the scan room while the magnet is energized
    b. The fire service should be allowed immediate access to an MR machine on fire due to the risk of explosion and the spread of fire to the rest of the hospital
    c. A 'quench' must be initiated as an emergency to switch off a resistive magnet in the event of a fire or cardiac arrest
    d. Oxygen cylinders should never be taken near an MR machine
    e. It is possible for a patient to become trapped against the MR machine by a ferrous metal object brought into the room

9. Magnetic Resonance Imaging: Answers

1a. True *

Spin angular momentum is an intrinsic property of an atom; those with equal numbers of protons and neutrons have no net spin and so no magnetic moment. With only a single proton, hydrogen has a large magnetic moment.

1b. True

This is known as the Larmor frequency and is unique for each element. The frequency varies with magnetic field strength and very slightly depending on what substance the proton is contained within.

1c. False

Although all of the hydrogen atoms will be affected, nearly as many will run anti-parallel, or in the opposite alignment to the field.

1d. False

It is the population difference between 'spin up' and 'spin down' states when subject to a strong magnetic field that produces the NMR signal. At room temperature in a 1 T magnet, the population differs by two for every one million nuclei involved.

1e. True

However, as this vector is in alignment with the magnetic field, it cannot be detected. By applying RF energy to the protons, their net magnetism can be altered into the x,y plane lying perpendicular to the static magnetic field (m_{xy}); this provides the signal for MRI.

2a. True **

The protons comprising hydrogen nuclei are most useful for medical imaging because they are so prevalent in the human body.

2b. True

C-13, O-17, F-19 and P-31 can all be used for MRI. At present imaging using anything other than protons is mainly for research purposes.

2c. False

Approximately half the protons will align 'spin up' and half will be 'spin down'. At 1 T approximately two extra protons out of every million will align spin up, and this difference accounts for the 'detectable' protons that allow the formation of the MR image.

2d. False

In the resting state the m_{xy} will be the sum of all the individual out of phase vectors pointing in random directions and thus will be equal to 0.

2e. False

A 1 T field is approximately 20 000 times greater than the earth's field strength of 50 μT.

3a. False ***

The z-axis is in line with the field. To enable creation of an MR signal, an RF pulse is applied which tips the net magnetic vector.

3b. False

Signal increases with static field strength.

3c. False
Increased PD (number of protons per unit volume) will give an increased signal.

3d. False
A coil can act in both transmit and receive modes, but not simultaneously.

3e. True
Water protons form the basis of most MRI, but protons are also very prevalent in fat.

4a. True ***
The signal is only detectable following the application of RF energy.

4b. True
The application of RF photons at the Larmor frequency will energize the hydrogen protons, causing them to precess in time with one another; this creates a signal which is detectable.

4c. False
A 180° pulse is enough energy to reverse the net magnetic vector. A 90° pulse is half as energetic (note this is the total energy of the pulse).

4d. False
Following an RF pulse, those protons in phase and creating a detectable MR signal will immediately begin to dephase due to T2 relaxation, and field inhomogeneities and the signal will rapidly diminish.

4e. False
It also depends on the field strength, RF pulse flip angle and also – to an extent depending on the pulse sequence timings used – on T1 and T2 relaxation processes and magnetic field inhomogeneities. With a higher field strength more protons are initially spin up.

5a. True *****
For hydrogen nuclei at 1 T it is approximately 42.6 MHz. It is proportional to field strength, and is also slightly affected by the substance it is in. The Larmor frequency for hydrogen within fat and water is very slightly different, which is the cause for chemical shift artefact.

5b. False
Photons with the same frequency as the Larmor frequency have the correct energy ($E = hf$) to cause the magnetic vector of a single proton to flip from spin up to spin down. At 1 T this is approximately 0.2 μeV. This frequency lies within the radio-wave end of the electromagnetic spectrum, which is why there is no ionizing radiation in MRI.

5c. False
A 180° pulse has approximately twice the number of photons, but the photons still all have to match the Larmor frequency and thus have the same energy.

5d. True
An initial 90° RF pulse flips the net magnetic vector such that it lies in the transverse xy plane, reducing the net m_z to 0. It also causes the individual protons to precess in phase and thus produces a detectable net m_{xy} rotating at the Larmor frequency.

5e. True

The signal used to generate the image is caused by the rotating magnetic vector inducing a current to flow in the RF coils in the same way that a dynamo works. This current is used to form the image.

6a. False ***

T1 recovery is in the longitudinal direction and is also known as spin–lattice relaxation. T1 is the time for 63% maximum recovery.

6b. True

Stronger magnetic fields hasten the precession, this lengthens T1.

6c. True

This occurs as they both have a short T1.

6d. True

T1-weighted images require a short TR and a short TE. Tissues with a short T1 will appear bright with these settings.

6e. True

Protons dephase faster than they realign with the static magnet.

7a. False ****

It is transverse relaxation.

7b. True

Tissues with a long T2 relaxation time give a high MR signal with T2 weighting. TE should ideally be of the order of the T2 relaxation time of the tissues of interest.

7c. False

CSF, urine, amniotic fluid and water all have long T2 and are therefore high signal. Blood flowing into the imaged slice after the initial 90° RF pulses does not produce signal.

7d. True

The difference is minimal, approximately 10 ms.

7e. True

This has most effect in solids which have a very short T2.

8a. False ***

Spin–spin relaxation leads to T2 decay through the transfer of energy between adjacent nuclei.

8b. False

T2* refers to free induction decay (FID); the combined effect of T2 relaxation and magnetic field inhomogeneities.

8c. False

This is true of T1. T2 is unaffected by magnet strength.

8d. True

If only a single 90° pulse is applied, the MR signal undergoes FID; true spin–spin relaxation is enhanced by magnetic field inhomogeneities. This situation is referred to as T2* and is generally countered using a 180° rephasing pulse.

8e. True

T2 is the time when 37% of the transverse magnetization remains. T1 is the time at which 63% of the longitudinal signal has recovered.

9a. False ****

T1 recovery is also known as spin−lattice relaxation and describes the recovery of the longitudinal magnetization of its equilibrium value along z, with associated loss of energy to the sorrounding lattice. T2 decay is spin−spin relaxation and describes the dephasing of the m_{xy} vector due to the small fields caused by surrounding dipoles. An FID signal, however, has amplitude which depends on T2* relaxation. T2* is more rapid than T2 and includes the dephasing effects of magnetic field inhomogeneities.

9b. True

T2* is the decay caused by field inhomogeneities plus tissue relaxation. A further 180° RF pulse in SE sequences helps to reduce the effect of field inhomogeneities by rephasing the m_{xy} and thus tissues show a true T2 signal.

9c. True

Conversely, T2 is the time for the m_{xy} to fall to 37% of its value.

9d. True

Fat and large molecules such as proteins in fluid are effective at removing energy in spin−lattice relaxation; this shortens T1. However, in solids, where water is more tightly bound, T1 relaxation becomes less efficient and T1 lengthens.

9e. False

In water, where molecules are moving around very rapidly, dipole−dipole interactions are very brief, making T2 relaxation less efficient, leading to a long T2.

10a. False ****

Due to the difficulty in switching instantaneously between RF transmit and receive, an echo of the FID is usually formed.

10b. False

The rephasing pulse is of 180°.

10c. True

A time TE/2 after the initial 90° pulse, the rephasing pulse is applied. A useful analogy to this is to imagine a running race suddenly reversed; the fastest runners (spins) are now at the back, and the slowest are at the front. Following a further time T, these differences will cancel out since the faster runners will catch the slower. At this point the net transverse magnetization peaks and since there has been a delay (TE) from RF transmission, there is plenty of time for the coils to be switched to receive.

10d. False

Although the magnet is currently unavoidably imperfect, the presence of the patient in the scanner always creates local field inhomogeneities.

10e. True

TE is time to echo and is double the time between 90° and 180° pulses. With a longer TE, there is more time for T2 decay to occur.

11a. True ***

This is one of the reasons it is utilized.

11b. True

The patient becomes very slightly magnetized and distorts the static field.

11c. False

Rephasing removes the effect T2*, but it takes time (TE) to achieve this. During this time, true T2 decay has occurred.

11d. True

They dephase very quickly, however, which necessitates the 180° rephasing pulse.

11e. True

The signal is registered at TE when maximum rephasing has occurred, i.e. the length of time that dephasing occurred prior to application of the 180° pulse is equal to the time needed for rephasing.

12a. False ****

A T1-weighted image would typically have a short TR of 300–800 ms and a short TE of 15 ms.

12b. False

These parameters would be typical of a T1-weighted image. A T2 would have a long TR of about 1000–2000 ms to eliminate the effect of T1 recovery and a long TE of 90–140 ms to allow the different T2 decay signals to become apparent.

12c. True

Water has a very long T2 relaxation time.

12d. False

Cortical bone and air appear dark on all MR weightings as they have very few protons.

12e. True

Inversion recovery sequences can reduce the signal from a certain type of tissue by timing a 90° pulse to occur when the m_z is 0 for that tissue type. STIR uses this to suppress the signal from fat. Fluid attenuated inversion recovery (FLAIR) uses this to suppress the signal from water.

13a. False **

Signal strength in a given tissue depends not only on the PD but also on the T1 and T2, via the pulse sequence used and its timing parameters. High signal is achieved with a high PD, a longer TR (relative to T1; means more protons have recovered prior to repeat), and a shorter TE (relative to T2; means less T2 decay has occurred). These features are balanced for image weighting.

13b. False

This would provide a PD-weighted image.

13c. False

With long T1, water is low signal on T1-weighted sequences, since less recovery of longitudinal magnetization can occur relative to tissue in a given TR.

13d. True

The PD of varying tissues is very similar due to their equally high water content.

13e. False

It is not possible for TE to be longer than TR.

14a. False ****

This is commonly how it is used but in MR any plane can be used for slice selection.

14b. True

Once the frequency encoding gradient is applied, the protons of interest will precess with frequency that varies according to their position along the gradient. Spatial localization is then achieved by identifying particular frequencies.

14c. False

Each step in the phase encoding direction takes TR. With perhaps 256 steps, the time to image each slice is 256 × TR. Only in 'single shot' techniques, such as EPI, can an entire slice be acquired in one TR.

14d. True

Assuming the frequency bandwidth of the excitation RF pulse is the same; slices could also be made thinner by use of a narrower bandwidth RF pulse with the same gradient.

14e. False

The raw data from each TR are stored in a K-space. This is a spatial frequency domain. 2D Fourier transformation of the entire K-space dataset produces the image.

15a. True ****

Slice select gradient together with the RF bandwidth determines the thickness of slice selected.

15b. False

Phase encoding data take a lot longer to accumulate. Traditionally, each phase encoding step takes time TR. Modern techniques can allow collection of several phase encoding steps in each TR, but phase encoding is still the time limiting factor in MR.

15c. False

The periphery of the K-space contains data relating to spatial resolution. The centre contains data for high signal intensity.

15d. True

Increasing the gradient of the applied field also reduces slice thickness. Thin slices produce better anatomical detail, but have a lower SNR.

15e. True

This can cause the wrap-around artefact in the phase encoding direction.

16a. True ****

This dual-echo imaging technique (two sets of images, one proton density weighted and one T2-weighted) can be produced from a single pulse sequence.

16b. True

The standard SE sequence is preceded by a 180° pulse. This allows more time for differences in the longitudinal relaxation of spins to become apparent.

16c. False

STIR is a method of fat suppression. Following a 180° inversion pulse, a 90° pulse is applied when longitudinal magnetization of fat has recovered to the point where it passes through the origin ($M_z = O$), i.e. fat has no signal. Thus only water protons are stimulated and the signal from fat has been suppressed.

16d. False

Gradient echo rephases spins faster than SE can through an initial reversal of the frequency encoding signal; however, magnet inhomogeneities are not countered by this means and the image is still T2*-weighted.

16e. False

EPI is a fast technique where an entire slice can be obtained in under 100 ms. A single excitation undergoes multiple rephasing of signal; resolution is usually lower, for example, 64×64 matrix, but its speed makes it useful for functional imaging.

17a. True ****

GRE uses a reduced strength RF pulse and short tip angle allowing for a short TR.

17b. False

Multiple phase encoding acquisition can be carried out in this way as phase encoding is the time-limiting factor in an SE sequence.

17c. True

It does this by inverting the protons with an initial 180° pulse which is then followed rapidly by a 90° pulse. The fat recovers quicker than other soft tissues and the 90° pulse is timed to occur when the fat signal is zero, thereby suppressing the signal from fat in the image.

17d. False

Pulse sequences can be adapted to aquire a series of slices, either sequentially or in an interleaved fashion, exciting and collecting data from a number of slices before returning to the first after time TR.

17e. True

Diffusion shows high signal from tissues which have abnormal proton movement within tissue water.

18a. True *****

Using a reduced tip angle allows m_z to recover more quickly so that TR can be reduced and still produce adequate signal strength.

18b. True

Taking several sets of phase encoded data per excitation can greatly reduce the time of the scan.

18c. False

This describes multi-slice CT. Multi-slice MR excites and collects echoes from other slices during the remainder of TR before returning to the first slice.

18d. False

Blood flowing into the region normally appears bright as it has not previously been excited and therefore has a full m_z available for excitation. This can give it a stronger signal than surrounding tissues which will have been previously excited. In contrast-enhanced MRA, the gadolinium agent greatly shortens the T1 of blood, making it appear bright in a T1 acquisition.

18e. False

Gadolinium contrast shortens both the T1 and T2 times. This would have the effect of a darker area on T2. Imaging after gadolinium is almost always using T1 weighting, and areas of uptake appear bright on T1.

19a. True ***

Commonly gadolinium; it has seven unpaired electrons, making it strongly paramagnetic. In a magnetic field, paramagnetic agents create their own alternating magnetic field, which encourages relaxation in neighbouring protons, shortening both T1 and T2. Ferromagnetic agents (iron oxide compounds) decrease the MR signal to provide negative contrast.

19b. False

Flowing blood is high signal because protons entering the slice plane are previously unexcited and therefore more signal is available for excitation than in surrounding stationary tissue which has not fully recovered from previous pulses.

19c. True

Ischaemic or infarcted tissue has lost cell integrity; the resultant oedema restricts diffusion.

19d. True

With four of its six outer electrons unpaired, deoxyhaemoglobin is strongly paramagnetic while oxygenated haemoglobin is, like most other soft tissues, diamagnetic. In active brain cells there is a net decrease in deoxyhaemoglobin; this can be detected with very rapid imaging providing a map of neuronal activity.

19e. True

For example, the Larmor frequency for hydrogen differs by 192–220 Hz if fat and water are compared in a 1.5 T magnet.

20a. False **

On SE slow flowing (e.g. venous) blood appears bright as previously unexcited blood enters the scan plane and is more affected by the 90° pulse and thereby produces a larger echo.

20b. False

GRE produces high signal in flowing blood without the need for contrast.

20c. True

Movement artefact is more apparent in the phase encoding direction as each phase encoding step is separated by time TR.

20d. False

Calcification produces no signal in MRI. This phenomenon can occur in CT angiography, however, when high attenuation calcium masks a stenosis in a contrast-filled vessel.

20e. False

Turbulent flow produces a loss of coherence and results in a low signal area.

21a. False ****

Movement is especially problematic in the phase encoded direction since each step is separated by time TR.

21b. True

This is the basis for MR angiography.

21c. False

Ferromagnetic objects decrease the MR signal causing a localized signal void.

21d. True

This makes subtle differences in the Larmor frequency less relevant to spatial encoding.

21e. False

Wrap-around occurs if the tissues which have been excited extend beyond the FOV. Phase encoding then inaccurately places the representative signal for these tissues within the image matrix.

22a. True ****

This occurs at the interface between tissue and fat. Fat has a slightly higher resonant frequency and this means it is erroneously allocated to a pixel located further up the gradient. This produces a black or white band at the fat–tissue interface.

22b. False

Chemical shift is more pronounced at higher field strength. Increasing the bandwidth can reduce this artefact.

22c. False

Ferrous metal implants distort or black out the surrounding areas. Streak artefact is seen in CT scanning.

22d. True

The sequence is triggered by the R-wave and TR equals the R–R interval.

22e. False

Aliasing or wrap-around results from the FOV being too small.

23a. False ***

Chemical shift artefact occurs as different tissues have very slightly different Larmor frequencies, e.g. fat compared with water. This difference is taken advantage of in the Dixon method of chemical shift imaging.

23b. False

Chemical shift is apparent in the frequency encoding direction. As the resonant frequencies of fat and water protons are very slightly different, their relative positions are slightly incorrect in the image in the frequency encoding direction. This can cause apparent overlap and gaps between fat and soft tissue in the image. Where the frequencies overlie one another there will be a white band, and to the other side of the structure where there is a gap of frequencies there will be a black band. Essentially it is as if the fatty or fluid object is cut out and shifted across the background by a short distance because the change in frequency causes the scanner to register it as a change in position.

23c. True

Odd appearances of toes behind the heel etc. can interfere with the picture. Increasing the FOV can help to solve this problem.

23d. True

Movement artefacts are therefore only really seen in the phase encoding direction, even if the direction of movement of the object is in the frequency encoding direction.

23e. True

Ferrous objects significantly increase the local field inhomogeneities and degrade the image or even black it out completely by rapidly dephasing m_{xy}. Gradient echo sequences are more susceptible to this than SE. This effect is sometimes of an advantage, however, as haemoglobin is slightly ferrous and a surrounding black area can help to indicate its presence.

24a. False ***

Spatial resolution is independent of the physical size of coil elements. However, using coils with multiple elements in a parallel imaging mode can allow improvements in spatial resolution. Dedicated surface or small loop coils placed directly over the anatomy of interest may greatly improve the SNR and therefore indirectly improve resolution by allowing a finer image matrix to be used.

24b. True

Being closer to the patient means less noise is detected.

24c. False

SNR is proportional to the square root of voxel volume. Therefore larger voxels improve SNR. However, this is balanced against a lower spatial resolution.

24d. False

If this were true there would be no need for the many other sequences available.

24e. False

A daily measurement of SNR would provide a good overall check of system performance. Only for special applications would frequent tests of magnet homogeneity be required (for example, MR spectroscopy).

25a. False ****

Thinner slices increase spatial resolution because the partial volume effect is less.

25b. False

The majority of noise is from the presence of the patient in the magnet. Random thermal movement of the hydrogen atoms in the patient produce RF 'white noise'. A Faraday cage in the walls of the scanning room reduces external RF noise.

25c. False

Gadolinium shortens the T1 of the adjacent hydrogen nuclei; its molecules do not emit a MR signal.

25d. True

Higher field strengths do increase the signal, however, the extent to which this occurs depends on the pulse sequence used, since T1 will be increased.

25e. False

Any pulse sequence will contain an element of both T1 and T2 weighting. However, deliberately introducing both T1 and T2 weighting (i.e. long TE, short TR) is unlikely to be useful as the contrasts produced by each type of weighting tend to cancel each other out.

26a. False ***

Noise in plain X-ray and CT is predominantly due to quantum mottle. Noise in MR is predominantly due to induction in the RF coils caused by random thermal motion of particles in the tissues of the patient.

26b. False

High signal increases the SNR, and therefore makes the noise less apparent. Noise is most apparent in areas of low signal intensity.

26c. False

Decreasing the voxel size would decrease the SNR unless another parameter was also altered to compensate for this.

26d. True

Increasing TR would allow more T1 recovery and therefore more m_z available to tip. Decreasing TE decreases the amount of decay of m_{xy}.

26e. True

Doubling N_{ex} would increase the SNR but double the scan time.

27a. False ***

The main magnet could also be a permanent magnet or a resistive electromagnet; these only provide strengths of up to 0.3 T and 0.5 T, respectively. Superconducting electromagnets can achieve up to 10 T in a small bore.

27b. False

Cooling is required to near $0°K$ or $-273°C$ (absolute zero).

27c. False

These are usually turned off at the end of the day; superconducting magnets are designed to remain on throughout their lifetime.

27d. False

The main magnetic field must be stable. Gradients are produced by separate, lower field strength gradient coils.

27e. True

Z is horizontal for tunnel-type magnets and vertical for many open magnets.

28a. False ***

It takes several hours for the current in the coil to build up. Once the unit is superconducting, the supply is shorted and the current continues to flow within the magnet without drawing any further external current.

28b. True

If the cooling fails, the system will rapidly heat up due to a loss of superconductivity causing resistive heat losses in the magnet windings. This results in rapid boil-off of liquid helium.

28c. False

The Faraday cage is a wire mesh that serves to screen the scanner from external RF interference.

28d. False
This is inverse square law which applies to radiation exposure. Modern MRI scanner static fields generally fall-off more rapidly due to active shielding.

28e. False
Surface coils give better SNR and/or resolution for near-surface tissues but less uniformity. The signal from near to the surface coil is much brighter than on the opposite side of the FOV.

29a. False **
The strength of a 0.5 T magnet is 0.5 T. It does not matter what type of magnet is producing it. However, only superconducting magnets are really capable of producing fields of above 0.5 T. Resistive magnets are limited to approximately 0.5 T by heating effects, and permanent magnets are only made in field strengths up to about 0.3 T.

29b. False
The term paramagnetic is used to describe how some molecules behave within a magnetic field; gadolinium is an example of a paramagnetic substance.

29c. False
A permanent magnet cannot be shut down at all. A resistive magnet may be shut down rapidly by switching off the power. A superconducting magnet may be shut down but only very slowly if a quench is to be avoided. In a true emergency the helium is released raising the temperature of the magnet and thus removing the superconducting properties. This has the effect of rapidly reducing the field strength, but even this method is not as fast as switching off a resistive magnet and can prove very expensive and damaging to the equipment.

29d. True
This reduces field inhomogeneities and thus allows better images to be obtained.

29e. True
This is most commonly seen in spinal MRI with surface coils along the back giving very detailed images of the spine.

30a. False **
The RF coils can act as both transmitter and receiver. The delay in switching is one reason for creating signal echoes.

30b. False
It is the rapid switching on and off of gradient coils that creates the noise in MRI.

30c. False
Surface coils are only effective to a depth in the patient equal to the diameter of the coil; therefore they are generally used for detailed imaging of specific, usually superficial, structures (e.g. lumbar spine).

30d. True
When used in parallel imaging mode, these coils each receive independent signal within the same imaging sequence. The data are then combined and knowledge of the spatial sensitivities of the individual coil elements can be used to cut down the number of phase encoding steps required.

30e. True

This is of particular import for phased array coils where the amplitude needs to be carefully controlled.

31a. True **

Elongated objects with a ferrous component (for example, a spanner) will tend to align themselves with the magnetic field, experiencing a strong torque force.

31b. True

Rapid change in the gradient fields causes vibration of the coils, hence acoustic noise in excess of 90 dB. Damage to hearing can occur over 90 dB, therefore hearing protection is mandatory.

31c. False

Significant fringe fields can extend for up to several metres from the magnet bore. Within the controlled area there is a risk of damage to, or interference with the function of, sensitive equipment or personal effects. Within the inner controlled area (which contains the 3 mT field contour and is usually defined to be the scan room), there is a risk of the projectile effect.

31d. False

Induced currents are the main concern with gradient fields; these can lead to nerve stimulation. RF fields can cause heating.

31e. True

A quench causes release of the liquid helium coolant; at room temperature it will return to a large volume of gas which can displace oxygen from the room.

32a. True ***

These are based on both Health Protection Agency advice and international guidelines (ICNIRP). They also implement European directives.

32b. False

They should not be in an area where the stray fields may be greater than 0.5 mT.

32c. False

Ethics approval is always required if research involves humans. Special approval may be required if using field strengths greater than 2 T.

32d. False

Firmly implanted metalwork will not usually move in the magnetic field. The presence of a ferromagnetic aneurysm clip is a contraindication.

32e. False

Gadolinium is not iodine-based. Patients with renal impairment may be at a small risk of developing nephrogenic systemic fibrosis.

33a. False ***

Although torque of metallic objects embedded in sensitive tissues is a concern, the safety issue with pacemakers is not only that they or the wires will move, but primarily that the MR scanner will interfere with the electrical function of the pacemaker.

33b. False

Non-ferrous metal foreign bodies that are firmly fixed in place such as joint prostheses are generally safe to scan, although they may be subject to heating and can degrade image quality. Ferrous foreign bodies such as aneurysm clips and especially metal eye foreign bodies can cause significant injury if movement is caused by the strong magnetic field. Any history of eye injury such as metal grinding should lead to an X-ray of the orbits to exclude metal foreign bodies before the MR scan is commenced.

33c. False

Initial patient screening should ideally be performed well before the patient arrives at the department. In a more acute setting this should be performed outside the controlled area; only those who have been screened (staff and patients) should ever enter the controlled area.

33d. True

Although currently there are no legal requirements limiting magnetic exposure, and no ill effects have been documented in humans, guidelines recommend avoiding MR in pregnant patients if possible and no greater than 2.5 T exposure if deemed necessary.

33e. False

SAR is the amount of RF power in watts per kg deposited, and is used to calculate safe heating levels given the patient's weight. No ionizing radiation is used in MRI.

34a. True ***

The controlled area in an MRI suite must contain the 0.5 mT field limit.

34b. False

Pacemakers are entirely restricted from the controlled area; this precludes the scanning of such patients.

34c. True

These are international guidelines (ICNIRP) upon which the UK MHRA guidelines are based. Normal scanning should be less than 2 T, with 'careful medical supervision' above this level; imaging greater than 4 T is restricted to research. Different limits are suggested for extremities including the head.

34d. False

The majority of prostheses are now non-ferrous and this would be checked carefully by MR staff prior to scanning. Large prostheses are generally firmly sited and movement is not a concern. Local RF heating and image distortion do need to be considered.

34e. True

This occurs through the induction of eddy currents; peripheral nerve stimulation may cause muscular contraction, but ventricular fibrillation is possible.

35a. False ***

The changing gradient fields can induce currents in tissue causing peripheral nerve stimulation. At higher rates of change of gradients muscle stimulation and even ventricular fibrillation can occur.

35b. False

The RF field can cause heating. If cables or metallic objects are in contact with skin, burning can occur.

35c. False

The RF field may cause an increase in temperature but the primary concern is that these objects will rotate to align with the magnetic field causing damage to the surrounding tissues. Anyone with a possible history of metal fragments in their eye (e.g. occupational exposure) should have an orbital X-ray prior to the MRI.

35d. False

This is not the case. All ferromagnetic materials should be removed before entering the controlled area; lead would not prevent the magnetic attraction of such objects.

35e. False

SAR is the RF energy deposited per mass of tissue and expressed in Wkg^{-1}. Restricting the SAR to 1.0 should not raise body temperature by more than 0.5°C.

36a. True ***

While the magnet is still on, a resuscitation team that may not know the risks of the magnetic field can present a risk to the patient or themselves. They may be carrying metal items that might harm the patient, and/or they might be at risk themselves through having a pacemaker or metal foreign bodies in their eyes, etc. The patient should be moved on an MR compatible trolley to a resuscitation area outside of the controlled area.

36b. False

There should not be any significant risk of explosion of the MR machine; helium is an inert gas and therefore is not flammable. The fire service often carries a significant amount of metal objects, and a firefighter attached to metal breathing apparatus or equally worse a fire axe flying at high velocity towards the machine may cause significant injury. Non-ferrous carbon dioxide fire extinguishers should be available within the department.

36c. False

A significant advantage of a resistive magnet is that in an emergency it can be switched off almost immediately. The magnet would not be quenched for a cardiac arrest unless the patient was also trapped.

36d. False

Although many conventional oxygen cylinders are constructed from steel and are thus dangerous near high field strength magnets, non-ferrous MR safe oxygen cylinders can be obtained. Equipment that is MR-conditional (safe under specific field conditions) or MR-safe should be clearly marked as such, and any item that is not so marked should not be taken within the environs of the MR scanner.

36e. True

The movement of a heavy ferrous object towards the magnet bore is likely to cause injury if it traps a patient. The magnet should be switched off as soon as possible to allow the release of the patient or staff member. In a permanent magnet this may present a serious problem. Obviously, the best way to deal with this is to avoid the problem happening in the first place, hence the many safety checks to enter the MR suite.

1. Regarding atomic structure:
   a. Protons are approximately 2000 times heavier than electrons
   b. The atomic number of an element is equal to the number of protons plus neutrons
   c. Electron binding energy is greatest in the valence shell
   d. Valence shell electrons are concerned with the electrical properties of an element
   e. The maximum number of electrons in the K-shell is 4

2. Concerning electromagnetic radiation:
   a. The energy of a photon is directly proportional to the frequency
   b. Microwaves, X-rays, and gamma rays are examples of ionizing radiation
   c. Electromagnetic radiation always follows the inverse square law
   d. The beam intensity measured as energy fluence rate is measured as the sum of the energy of the photons per unit area per unit time
   e. A typical wavelength for diagnostic X-rays is 400 nm

3. In the clinical production of X-rays, the following are true:
   a. The energy of fast moving electrons striking a target is mostly converted to X-rays
   b. There are two electrical currents in the system
   c. High frequency X-ray generators provide a steady supply with approximately 10% ripple
   d. Characteristic X-rays from a tungsten target have energies of 58 and 68 keV
   e. A molybdenum target provides lower energy characteristic X-rays than a tungsten target

4. Interaction of X-rays with matter:
   a. X-rays are directly ionizing
   b. Following photoelectric absorption in soft tissue, characteristic radiation is released
   c. The photoelectric effect is less likely with higher energy X-rays
   d. K-edge filters ideally have a K-shell binding energy just above the mean X-ray beam energy
   e. X-rays ionize air

5. **Concerning Ionising Radiations Regulations 1999 (IRR99):**
   a. A controlled area is defined as an area where an employee is likely to be exposed to any amount of radiation
   b. When using mobile X-ray equipment, the controlled area is usually the area within 2 m of the patient and the X-ray tube
   c. The radiation protection advisor (RPA) is responsible for ensuring that work being performed is in accordance with local rules
   d. A 17-year-old employee who is likely to exceed three-tenths of the dose limit to the lens of the eye must be designated as a classified worker
   e. The employer must ensure that personal protective equipment (e.g. lead aprons) are being used appropriately

6. **Regarding the Ionising Radiation (Medical Exposure) Regulations (IR(ME)R):**
   a. Published in 2000 they were amended in 2002
   b. The Referrer and the Practitioner must be either a medical doctor or dentist
   c. The equipment service engineer is considered an Operator
   d. Compliance with the employer's procedures drawn up under IR(ME)R negates the need for ethics approval if undertaking research involving ionizing radiation
   e. Doses must be kept within diagnostic reference levels (DRLs)

7. **Radiation protection:**
   a. Irradiation of the pelvis in a pregnant female can never be justified
   b. Optimization of a procedure requires adequate quality assurance (QA)
   c. Dose limits for staff represent a good practice guide
   d. Patient dose limits are higher than those for the general public
   e. The annual effective dose limit for a trainee less than 18 years old is three-tenths that of an adult employee

8. **Regarding image quality:**
   a. Noise in an image can adversely affect both spatial resolution and contrast
   b. A high resolution image might have 15 lp/mm
   c. Quantum mottle is defined as $\sqrt{M}$, where M is the mean number of photons detected per pixel
   d. Noise increases with higher signal
   e. An increased kV reduces subject contrast

9. **Scatter:**
   a. For radiography in the chest and abdomen, there is less scatter radiation detected than transmitted primary beam
   b. Has less effect on the image with a lower kV
   c. Will lessen as grid ratio increases
   d. Is more efficiently eliminated with a moving grid
   e. An air gap is necessary if using a grid

10. **Focal spot:**
    a. A small target angle minimizes unsharpness
    b. It is not technically possible to create focal spots of less than 0.3 mm
    c. By rotating the anode a smaller effective focal spot is achieved
    d. The anode heel effect is greatest at the cathode side of the X-ray beam
    e. Focal spot size is assessed with an ionization chamber

11. **Quality assurance in radiography:**
    a. Beam kV may be assessed with a sensitometer
    b. The equipment supplier is responsible for ensuring that a QA programme is maintained for the life of the equipment
    c. Spatial resolution in fluoroscopy is assessed using a Leeds test object
    d. Monitors may be tested with 13 gradations of greyscale using standard Society of Motion Picture and Television Engineers (SMPTE) images
    e. Needs only to be performed yearly

12. **In mammography:**
    a. Useful target-filter combinations include molybdenum–rhodium, rhodium–rhodium, and rhodium–molybdenum
    b. The mean energy of X-rays used is in the range of 15 to 20 keV
    c. To utilize the anode–heel effect, the tube axis runs parallel to the chest wall
    d. Heat loading of the focal spot limits exposure time
    e. To assess risk, mean glandular dose is used instead of effective dose

13. **Film-based radiography:**
    a. X-ray film is more sensitive to light than to X-rays
    b. Caesium iodide (CsI) is the active ingredient in film which forms the latent image
    c. Processing occurs independently of temperature
    d. An optical density (OD) of 2 means 99% of light incident on the processed film is transmitted
    e. Film is no longer used in modern radiography

14. **Digital imaging:**
    a. Edge enhancement software improves spatial resolution but also increases noise
    b. DICOM is the industry standard in medical imaging and is shorthand for DIgital COMmunication
    c. Does not involve sampling
    d. With Fourier analysis fine structures have a high spatial frequency
    e. Aliasing occurs if the Nyquist frequency is not met

15. **Computed radiography (CR):**
    a. Requires entirely new equipment for a department changing from film–screen
    b. Utilizes photostimulable phosphors
    c. Is an entirely digital process
    d. Has a wide dynamic range
    e. Generally spatial resolution is less than with film–screen systems

16. **Digital radiography (DR):**
    a. Implies imaging is achieved directly from the plate
    b. Can be direct or indirect, where indirect uses phosphors
    c. The detective quantum efficiency for DR is roughly doubled that of CR and film–screen
    d. The number of pixels in the image can be increased by choosing a smaller field of view (FOV)
    e. In general, overexposed images are immediately apparent when viewed

17. **Image intensifier design:**
    a. The input screen has a diameter approximately 50 times that of the output screen
    b. The input screen converts X-ray photons to light; the light photons are then accelerated across to the output screen
    c. The input screen is maintained at a negative voltage
    d. The image on the output screen is inverted relative to the input screen
    e. Within the intensifier an inert gas such as argon is used for stability

18. **Regarding the image intensifier:**
    a. The sequence of events in image formation is as follows: X-ray photons to light, light to electrons, electrons back to light
    b. Gain refers to the increased resolution achieved
    c. Intensification occurs as a product of flux gain and minification gain
    d. Magnification reduces intensification
    e. Automatic brightness control follows pre-programmed curves

19. **Image quality in fluoroscopy:**
    a. Continuous fluoroscopy is actually pulsed
    b. The patient entrance surface dose rate may be up to $200 \ mGymin^{-1}$ to provide adequate image quality
    c. The quantum sink in fluoroscopy is the number of X-ray photons incident at the input screen
    d. Using an X-ray field that extends beyond the edge of the patient may result in a loss of image quality
    e. An image intensifier would not work properly in a room adjacent to a magnetic resonance (MR) scanner

20. **Using digital subtraction angiography (DSA):**
    a. Eliminates the need for contrast agents
    b. The pixel value of the mask image is subtracted from subsequent images
    c. Pixel shifting allows correction for movement in portions of the image when other areas are static
    d. Can be used in realtime
    e. Leads to an increase in noise

21. **Flat plate detectors for fluoroscopy:**
    a. Use the same technology as DR
    b. Have improved spatial resolution when compared with the image intensifier
    c. Often require magnification to maximize resolution
    d. Suffer from the same geometrical distortion as image intensifiers
    e. Remove the need for collimation

22. **Regarding the computed tomography (CT) image:**
    a. The CT number for fat is approximately 50
    b. Around 4000 levels of grey are generally possible in a CT image
    c. Windowing limits the visible grey scale to make tissue contrast more discernable to the human eye
    d. Voxel isotropy means neighbouring voxels have the same CT number
    e. A tissue detail with dimensions smaller than a voxel is only visible because of partial volume effects

23. **Equipment in CT:**
    a. Modern scanners are based on 4th generation design
    b. The anode–cathode axis lies parallel to the z-axis
    c. Thanks to slip ring technology, each 360° rotation of the gantry takes around 2 sec
    d. Focal spot heat capacity is approximately 4 MJ
    e. Detectors such as bismuth germinate are used

24. **CT image quality:**
    a. To ensure accurate CT numbers are produced the scanner must be calibrated to air, water and bone
    b. The maximum resolution achievable on current CT scanners is around 20 lp/mm
    c. Voxel noise is directly related to slice thickness
    d. Pitch has no effect on noise
    e. Noise is more apparent when using a narrower window width

25. Concerning CT artefacts:
a. Cardiac motion artefact can be reduced by administering drugs to slow the heart rate
b. Beam hardening can be partly corrected by using a copper bow-tie filter
c. Ring artefact is observed in patients with metal implants or jewellery
d. A faulty detector can result in wrap-around artefact on the reconstructed image
e. Thicker slices will give an increased likelihood of partial volume effect

26. Regarding CT scanning:
a. CT fluoroscopy is only possible since the advent of slip ring technology
b. Multi-slice CT scanners do not require the use of any beam filtration
c. Typically tube voltage is in excess of 140 kV
d. Solid-state detectors such as cadmium tungstate have greater detection efficiency than xenon gas ionization chambers
e. The acquisition time of a CT head scan using a helical scanner is typically in the region of 60 sec

27. Concerning radioactivity:
a. The number of decays per second will remain constant while a radionuclide is radioactive
b. Isotopes of an element have the same mass number but may have a different atomic number
c. Radionuclides are unstable nuclei that undergo spontaneous decay with the emission of radiation until reaching a stable state
d. The exact timing of the decay of an individual atom is determined by the chemical properties of that particular isotope
e. After eight half-lives, the radioactivity of a set amount of radioactive matter will have reduced by a factor of 64

28. Image formation with a gamma camera:
a. X and Y coordinates are determined by an array of photomultiplier tubes
b. Collimators are rarely used
c. Spatial resolution and sensitivity to gamma radiation cannot both be maximized in the same study
d. Scatter is reduced using the pulse height analyser
e. It is not possible for gamma rays to be detected with energy greater than that characteristic for the radionuclide

29. **Single photon emission computed tomography (SPECT):**
    a. Involves combining many images at different angles to produce a three-dimensional (3D) image
    b. Photon counts for the acquisition at each angle are much higher than a single image of planar radionuclide imaging
    c. Opposing views allow some correction of attenuation of gamma rays within the patient
    d. Is rapid enough to take an entire image within a single breath-hold
    e. Can be gated to image the heart

30. **Positron emission tomography (PET) and PET–CT:**
    a. PET scanners use a single detection plate which acquires about 60 images revolving around the patient
    b. Narrow lead or tungsten septa are used as a grid to limit the angle of incoming photons
    c. The most commonly used radionuclide in PET scanning is ^{99}Technetium metastable (Tc-99m)
    d. PET–CT image reconstruction includes a tissue correction algorithm based on the CT scan
    e. Fusion of PET and CT images most commonly involves combining a PET and a CT scan of the same patient taken up to six months apart

31. **Image quality in radionuclide imaging:**
    a. A defective photomultiplier tube will show as a linear defect on the image
    b. Electronic noise is the major limiting factor in radionuclide imaging quality
    c. A converging collimator can improve resolution for objects smaller than the area of the crystal
    d. Temporal resolution refers to blurring at the edges of the image
    e. Sodium iodide (NaI) is not used in PET imaging

32. **Regarding effective dose in nuclear medicine:**
    a. A Tc-99m bone scan is similar to a barium enema
    b. A cardiac scan with thallium-201 gives approximately five times the average natural annual background radiation in the UK
    c. A Tc-99m lung perfusion scan is the same as the annual whole body dose limit for a member of the public
    d. Effective dose can be reduced by encouraging the patient to drink plenty of water and empty their bladder
    e. In men, lead groin shields should be worn to reduce the dose to the gonads

33. **Safety when handling radionuclides:**
    a. It is good practice to vent air from the tip of the syringe into the atmosphere prior to administration
    b. Following administration of a radionuclide, patients should be restricted to a room with radiation shielding on the walls
    c. If contaminated, simple washing of hands is not sufficient
    d. Some waste can be dispersed to the environment
    e. Spills must be cleaned up immediately

34. **Sound waves in tissue:**
    a. The speed of sound in bone is faster than the speed of sound in soft tissue
    b. The speed of sound in most soft tissues is relatively independent of wavelength and frequency
    c. Acceleration of soft tissue particles by the ultrasound waves never reaches more than 10 g
    d. Ultrasound is an example of a transverse wave
    e. Ultrasound waves take approximately 7 μs to travel 1 cm

35. **Piezoelectric effect and probes:**
    a. The piezoelectric effect describes a property in which expansion or contraction of the piezoelectric element causes or is caused by an electric voltage
    b. Typical voltages applied within the ultrasound probe to transmit are in the region of 5–12 V.
    c. By applying different voltages to a linear array, the beam can be focused to a determined focal point
    d. An abdominal diagnostic ultrasound probe typically transmits for half the time it receives
    e. An ultrasound probe has a natural frequency with a wavelength of twice the thickness of the element

36. **Imaging techniques in ultrasound:**
    a. Sector scanning has a smaller 'footprint' than linear
    b. A greater depth of view can be achieved with a lower pulse repetition frequency (PRF)
    c. Contrast agents work because of their high density
    d. 3D imaging in ultrasound compiles several 2D slices
    e. Harmonic imaging utilizes the first harmonic

37. **Regarding the use of Doppler:**
    a. If ultrasound waves are reflected from an object moving towards the probe, the frequency of these reflected waves will be increased
    b. Doppler shift is greater for faster moving objects
    c. Is best determined at 90° to a moving object
    d. Doppler shift frequencies are generally in the audible sound range
    e. Duplex scanning combines Doppler data with B-mode scan images

38. Concerning nuclear magnetic resonance within a uniform 1 T static field:
    a. Proton precession is around the axis of the main magnetic field
    b. Protons precess at a variable frequency
    c. The static field is approximately 2000 times stronger than the earth's magnetic field
    d. The Larmor frequency is not affected by magnetic field strength
    e. A radiofrequency (RF) pulse equalling half the resonant frequency will flip the net magnetization of the sample through 90° from the z-axis

39. Spin-echo (SE) and gradient recalled echo (GRE) sequences:
    a. An SE sequence involves a 180° RF pulse after the 90° pulse to bring the m_{xy} back into phase
    b. In a GRE sequence dephasing of the M_{xy} due to inhomogeneities in the field is eliminated by a rephasing gradient
    c. Spoiled gradient echo deliberately introduces gradients and/or RF pulses to dephase the m_{xy}
    d. In SE the echo is obtained at a time to echo (TE) of twice the time between the 90 and 180° RF pulses
    e. GRE sequences typically have a very long TE

40. Spatial encoding:
    a. During slice selection a wider RF bandwidth for the same magnetic field gradient will reduce the thickness of slice selected
    b. During slice selection a greater magnetic field gradient for the same RF bandwidth will reduce the thickness of slice selected
    c. Information obtained from steep phase encode gradients forms the high spatial frequency resolution part of K-space
    d. The echo is obtained while the phase encoding gradient is switched on
    e. The phase encoding information is obtained in a series of steps each with a different amplitude phase encoding gradient

10. Mock Examination: Answers

1a. True ***

Protons and neutrons have a relative mass of 1, electrons have a relative mass of 0.0054.

1b. False

Atomic number is equal to the number of protons; mass number is equal to the number of protons plus neutrons.

1c. False

The valence shell is the outermost electron shell. Being furthest from the nucleus, attraction is weaker and so binding energy is lower.

1d. True

A loose valence shell electron in metals enables conductivity.

1e. False

The maximum is 2.

2a. True ***

Energy = hf, where h is Plank's constant.

2b. False

Microwaves are low frequency electromagnetic radiation, and the energy is not sufficient to produce ionization of water. X-rays and gamma rays are ionizing.

2c. False

The inverse square law only applies to a point source for electromagnetic radiation. While the focal spot is technically not a point source, it is small enough that the inverse square law can be applied with reasonable accuracy.

2d. True

Energy fluence is the sum of the energies. Photon fluence is the number of photons.

2e. False

This is the wavelength for blue light. X-rays have a wavelength of 1 nm or less.

3a. False ****

99% of the incident electron energy is converted to heat, the rest to X-rays.

3b. True

One is the tube potential used to accelerate electrons (high kV, low current), the other flows through the filament to liberate electrons (low kV, high current).

3c. False

Ripple is generally no greater than 2%.

3d. True

Characteristic energy values are equal to the difference in binding energy of the electron shells involved.

3e. True

For molybdenum, K_α photons have energy of 17.5 keV, while K_β have energy of approximately 20 keV. This compares with energies of 58 and 68 keV for tungsten.

4a. False **

X and gamma rays are indirectly ionizing; the secondary electrons (photoelectrons or those reflected in the Compton effect) form ion pairs along their path through a material. By contrast, alpha and beta particles ionize directly.

4b. True

This is of very low energy and usually absorbed immediately, often with the release of a further Auger electron.

4c. True

The photoelectric effect is inversely proportional to E^3.

4d. False

Ideally just below the mean beam energy.

4e. True

This is the principle behind an ionization chamber.

5a. False ***

A controlled area is defined as an area where an employee may potentially be exposed to three-tenths of any dose limit.

5b. True

It is not practical to assign an entire ward as a controlled area.

5c. False

This is the responsibility of the RPS.

5d. False

An individual under 18 years of age cannot be classified.

5e. True

The employee has a responsibility to use protective equipment as required by the employer. However, the employer would be in breach of the regulation if he allowed a member of staff to work with ionizing radiation without taking the required precautions.

6a. False **

The regulations were amended in 2006.

6b. False

Both the Referrer and the Practitioner must be registered health-care professionals and must be entitled to carry out those roles by the employer.

6c. True

The Operator is a broad role covering anyone involved in the practical aspects of the examination.

6d. False

Ethics Committee approval is still required.

6e. False

DRLs are a requirement under IR(ME)R but are based on local dose audit. They represent the typical dose for an average-sized patient; larger patients, for example, are likely to receive doses in excess of the DRL.

7a. False ***

When justifying procedures, benefit needs to outweigh risk. The benefit to the pregnant female from an accurate diagnosis will sometimes be of greater importance than the risk to the fetus. Such decisions are made by the Practitioner under IR(ME)R.

7b. True

Optimization requires that doses are kept as low as is reasonably practicable (ALARP). QA ensures equipment works as expected.

7c. False

It is illegal to allow an employee to receive a dose in excess of any dose limit. Doses to staff arising from the use of medical radiations are generally well below these limits.

7d. False

Patients do not have dose limits; the principles of Justification and Optimization are used to minimize patient exposure.

7e. True

This amounts to an annual effective dose of 6 mSv.

8a. True ****

Noise reduces contrast in an image and this can reduce the spatial resolution, particularly for low contrast features.

8b. True

This is the current upper limit achievable with film–screen mammography.

8c. True

The most significant cause of noise in radiology is quantum mottle. This represents variability in the number of photons detected in each pixel. Noise is calculated as the square root of the mean of the number of photons.

8d. True

With more events detected (a higher signal), there would be more noise. The signal to noise ratio (SNR), however, would improve since the noise is now a smaller proportion of the whole signal, i.e. less variability.

8e. True

This is why mammography uses low kV.

9a. False ***

Even in a chest X-ray (CXR) where scatter is minimal, there will be four times more than primary radiation at the detector. In a lateral pelvis it can be up to nine times.

9b. True

Less scatter travels forward with lower kV, so less will be incident on the detector.

9c. True

Grid ratio is the depth of the grid inter-space channel over the width. The larger the ratio, the more efficient the grid; but a more efficient grid will also remove more of the primary beam (cut off).

9d. False

Moving grids are used to minimize visible grid lines on the image.

9e. False

An air gap is an alternative technique for removing scatter.

10a. True ***
The smaller the target angle, the smaller the effective focal spot size and thus the unsharpness is minimized.

10b. False
In macro-radiography, the focal spot size might be 0.1 mm. It is technically possible to create even smaller focal spot sizes; the limitation is tube heating.

10c. False
The effective focal spot size is the same with a rotating anode. It rotates to improve heat dissipation.

10d. False
The anode heel effect occurs due to the target being angled; X-rays arising deep in the target and being emitted on the anode side of the beam have further to travel through the target and so undergo more attenuation before leaving the tube.

10e. False
A star grid or pin-hole collimator can be used to measure focal spot size for QA purposes. Focal spot sizes should be within tolerances of 25–50% from their stated size.

11a. False ***
A sensitometer is a device for measuring the characteristic curve of a film–screen combination. A penetrameter is commonly used for measuring kV.

11b. False
This is the duty of the employer under IRR99.

11c. False
This is used for assessing contrast; a line-pair test object is used for spatial resolution.

11d. True
The SMPTE test pattern grades in 10% increments from zero (black) to 100% (white). In addition, 5% and 95% are included in the scale and these should be distinguishable to the human eye if the monitor is calibrated properly, and viewing conditions optimized.

11e. False
Although some tests are carried out yearly, many are carried out much more frequently (up to daily).

12a. False ****
In order of mean energy, useful combinations include; molybdenum–molybdenum, molybdenum–rhodium, rhodium–rhodium and tungsten–rhodium. A rhodium–molybdenum combination would exclude rhodium characteristic rays because their energy is greater than the K-edge of molybdenum.

12b. True
Bremsstrahlung radiation has a mean energy that is about 50% of the tube voltage. However, in mammography the photon energy is largely determined by the characteristic radiation. The characteristic energies of molybdenum are 17.4 and 19.6 keV while those of Rh are 20.2 and 22.8 keV.

12c. False
The tube axis needs to be perpendicular to the chest wall, with the cathode on the chest side of the patient. Due to the anode heel effect the higher doses will be on the chest wall side where the breast thickness is greater even when compression is applied.

12d. False
Heat loading limits the available current, thereby requiring an increase in exposure time; this in turn necessitates patient immobilization.

12e. True
Effective dose is not a meaningful dose quantity when a single organ or tissue is irradiated.

13a. True ***
There is an interaction rate of only 2% between X-rays and film. This is why we use intensification screens.

13b. False
The active ingredient in film is silver bromide. Processing donates electrons to the ionized silver which creates visible silver atoms.

13c. False
An increase in temperature will lead to an increased rate of reaction. Increased developer concentration has a similar effect.

13d. False
OD is on a logarithmic scale; 0 = 100% light transmission, 1 = 10%, 2 = 1%, 3 = 0.1%. A normally exposed film has an OD of 1.

13e. False
At the time of writing, film is still used; particularly in mammography where the spatial resolution is higher than with digital systems and also in dental radiology.

14a. True ***
High pass spatial filtering incorporates a proportion of the difference between neighbouring pixels into each pixel; edges are therefore exaggerated, but so are fluctuations in signal (noise).

14b. False
DICOM is the industry standard but is an acronym of Digital Imaging and Communications in Medicine.

14c. False
Turning analogue data to an electronic signal always involves sampling. The higher the sampling frequency, the better the representation.

14d. True
Fourier analysis is a mathematical sampling technique used to convert spatial resolution to frequency.

14e. True
Nyquist criterion states that a signal must be sampled twice in every cycle to be accurately represented. If not, aliasing occurs.

15a. False ***
Only the 'plates' and the image processor are different. Tables, Bucky's and grids, etc. used for film–screen radiography are entirely compatible with CR.

15b. True
For example, barium flourohalide doped with europium.

15c. False

The X-ray intensity incident on the plate is first captured by the storage phosphor. An automatic plate reader incorporating a scanning laser beam then transforms this into a digital signal.

15d. True

Around 10 000:1

15e. True

CR is mostly limited by pixel size and so this may improve with time, but currently only achieves around 5 lp/mm for general radiography.

16a. True ****

Compare this with CR where a separate reader is required.

16b. True

Direct systems include amorphous selenium detectors whereas indirect systems incorporate a phosphor such as CsI to convert X-ray energy into light which is detected by an array of silicon diodes.

16c. True

Detective quantum efficiency (DQE) is the percentage of photons detected from the total number incident on the plate. Typically DR has a DQE of 65%, CR and film–screen 30%.

16d. False

Pixel number is determined by the number of detectors in the thin film transistor (TFT) array. A smaller FOV means less of these are utilized in the image.

16e. False

Unlike film–screen the wide dynamic range of both CR and DR means it is difficult to over-expose detectors in general use. Dose detector indicators are used as a safeguard to prevent excessive patient dose.

17a. False ****

Typically 10 to 15 times greater.

17b. False

Although X-rays are first converted to light photons in the CsI phosphor, these are then converted to electrons in the photocathode. It is the electrons that are accelerated to the output screen.

17c. True

This accelerates the electrons away through repulsion. The output screen acts as the anode.

17d. True

The focused electrons cross over.

17e. False

There is a vacuum within the intensifier.

18a. True ***

This process amplifies the signal.

18b. False

The gain refers to the increase in light signal from input to output screens. This enables visualization using smaller doses at the input screen. It has no effect on resolution.

18c. True

Flux gain caused by acceleration of the electrons increases signal by approximately 50 times, minification by around 100. The total brightness gain then is 5000.

18d. True

There is less minification gain as a smaller part of the image on the input screen is reproduced on the full area of the output screen.

18e. True

These curves adjust kV and mA as the detected signal varies at the input screen (with changing patient attenuation). Adjustments occur in a programmed fashion that depends on clinical application.

19a. True ***

At 25–30 frames per second the human eye cannot discern the pulses.

19b. False

Internationally accepted standards dictate that the dose rate should never exceed 100 mGymin^{-1}, commonly doses are around 25 mGymin^{-1}.

19c. False

Quantum sink refers to the step in the imaging process where the smallest number of photons or electrons is used to form the image. For an image intensifier the noise is determined by the number of photons detected by the input screen which is less than the number incident on it.

19d. True

This can produce veiling glare.

19e. True

Magnetic fields can cause geometrical distortion by distorting the paths of accelerated electrons. This may affect the image intensifier in an adjacent room.

20a. False ****

Without contrast, the vessels of interest would not be visible. DSA removes static background detail to make the contrast-filled vessels more apparent.

20b. False

The logarithms of the mask and post-contrast images are calculated and divided into each other prior to converting back to pixel values for display.

20c. False

Pixel shifting can only be applied to the full area of the image.

20d. True

There is a small delay in calculation but this is so short that the subtraction image is effectively viewed in realtime.

20e. False

By subtracting pixel values the total signal in the image is less, hence there is less noise ($\sqrt{\text{mean}}$). However, noise now forms a greater proportion of the total signal so SNR is less; i.e. the image appears noisier.

21a. True ***

Most flat plate detectors use indirect DR plates with CsI phosphors.

21b. True

Flat plates typically have resolution of about 3 lp/mm; image intensifiers are generally no better than 1.2 to 2 lp/mm for the largest FOV.

21c. False

These are digital images; magnification only enables the user to see detail more clearly because the image is magnified on the viewing monitor. The image resolution is unchanged as it is based on the pixel density of the receiver.

21d. False

With image intensifiers, pin cushion distortion is caused by the curved input screen while s-type distortion results from interference with the accelerated electrons; neither of these processes can therefore occur with flat plates.

21e. False

Doses should always be kept to a minimum and reducing field area invariably reduces patient (and staff) dose.

22a. False ***

Air is −1000, lung −800 to −300, fat −150 to −60, water is equal to 0, muscle is approximately 50 and bone is 500 to 1500.

22b. True

With 12-bit storage 4096 are possible (−1024 to 3071).

22c. True

The human eye can only cope with around 50 levels of grey.

22d. False

Voxel isotropy means its dimensions are the same in all three planes; this is necessary for true 3D reconstruction and was made possible with the advent of multi-slice CT.

22e. True

The CT number of any voxel represents the mean of all densities within it.

23a. False ***

Multi-detector CT scanners are based on the rotation of both X-ray source and detectors (3rd generation, rotate−rotate).

23b. True

This helps to avoid the anode heel effect in the plain of the detectors.

23c. False

Slip ring technology allows continuous rotation but with current design the rotation time may be 0.3 sec or less.

23d. True

This allows up to 90 sec of continuous scanning.

23e. True

These have a high detection efficiency and wide dynamic range.

24a. False ****

The scanner is only calibrated to air and water.

24b. False

CT resolution is currently about 20 lp/cm.

24c. False

Noise is directly related to the square root of slice thickness since thicker slices allow more photons per voxel and noise is calculated as the square root of the mean signal. Note that SNR will increase as slice thickness increases provided the tube current is not changed.

24d. False

This is true for single-slice as the number of photons used per voxel is unchanged. In multi-slice, however, use of fixed width interpolation means there are fewer photons sampled with an increased pitch, i.e. more noise.

24e. True

Remember that noise represents slight random variation in signal level. If the difference between minimum and maximum signal is reduced, this fluctuation becomes more apparent.

25a. True ***

Beta blockers are commonly used. The requirement for this may lessen with quicker scan times. In addition, scanning can be gated using electrocardiograms (ECGs).

25b. True

The beams travelling through the centre of the patient have been 'hardened' by passing through the periphery of the patient and therefore have a lower relative attenuation coefficient. A bow-tie filter provides progressively increased filtration to the outer rays of the fan beam.

25c. False

Metal causes streak artefact. Ring artefact is seen as a result of a faulty detector.

25d. False

Ring artefact is seen as a result of a faulty detector. Wrap-around is an artefact seen in MRI images.

25e. True

The partial volume effect is more likely with thicker slices.

26a. True ****

Slip ring technology enables the gantry to spin but maintains the high voltage supply to the X-ray generator and the transfer of data from the detectors.

26b. False

Beam filtration of 6 mm aluminium equivalent is typical. Copper bow-tie filters are also used to compensate for changing body cross-section.

26c. False

A typical tube voltage is 120 kV (range 80–140 kV).

26d. True

Solid-state detectors operate at a detection efficiency greater than 90%. Ionization chambers operate at approximately 60%.

26e. False

With multi-detector rows and helical scanning at rotation speeds of about 3 per second, significantly shorter scan times than this can be achieved.

27a. False ****
Activity diminishes exponentially until stability is reached.

27b. False
The atomic number determines the element. Isotopes differ in their mass number (number of protons and neutrons).

27c. True
Some of the energy released during this decay is harnessed for medical imaging.

27d. False
The half-life of an isotope is fixed, but the decay of individual nuclei is a stochastic event and therefore cannot be predicted; the shorter the half-life, the more likely it is to decay within a given time interval.

27e. False
It will have reduced by a factor of 2^8 (256).

28a. True **
Each light pulse in the crystal is detected by most, if not all, of the photomultipliers. The intensity detected in each allows localization of the light origin.

28b. False
Collimators are used to eliminate both primary radiation from regions outside the acceptance angle of the collimator aperture and secondary scattered radiation. The choice of collimator has implications for image resolution. In addition, collimators can also be used to magnify/minify an image.

28c. True
A high resolution collimator with a large number of small holes allows more accurate position determination but as less gamma radiation passes through, it is less sensitive. The converse is true for a high sensitivity collimator.

28d. True
A narrow window of acceptable gamma energies is chosen. This is centred on the energy of unattenuated gamma rays; scattered rays would have reduced energy and be excluded.

28e. False
Two simultaneous incident gamma rays would produce more light; the photomultipliers would thus detect a single, more energetic event. In addition there is some variability in photomultiplication; this could lead to a more energetic pulse than expected.

29a. True ***
One or several rotating gamma cameras collect up to 60 sets of images from around the patient.

29b. False
Photon counts for each angle are much lower than planar imaging.

29c. True
Obviously gamma rays from the centre or the far side of the patient will be attenuated more. By combining opposing views this effect can be averaged out.

29d. False

While CT has become this rapid, the speed of SPECT is limited by the activity of radiopharmaceutical given to the patient. Approximately 3 million counts are needed to produce most SPECT scans, and this may take 30 min or more. Consequently movement artefact is a significant problem.

29e. True

Although the total scan time may be quite long, gating allows the data from each part of the cardiac cycle to be added together, and a short clip of cardiac function taken as an average of many heart beats.

30a. False ****

This would be more typical for SPECT. PET scanners have to detect photons arriving simultaneously 180° apart and are therefore normally built as a complete ring of detectors around the patient.

30b. True

This helps reduce false events of two photons from separate events arriving at the same time and thus giving the appearance of an event in the incorrect place.

30c. False

Tc-99 m is a gamma ray emitter commonly used in planar nuclear imaging such as bone scans and ventilation perfusion scans. Fluorine-18, used as fluorine deoxyglucose (FDG), is the most commonly used in PET.

30d. True

The CT scan gives information that can be used to correct for the tissue attenuation of the gamma rays, giving a more accurate image.

30e. False

Software is available to fuse separately acquired PET data and a normal CT scan, but because of patient positioning and movement this is prone to error. A combined PET–CT scanner produces images with minimal delay between examinations with identical patient positioning; the correlation between the two is far more accurate.

31a. False ****

Detector uniformity is checked using a flood field. A defective photomultiplier will show a round area of low signal; a linear defect indicates a crack in the crystal.

31b. False

Statistical variation in signal from one pixel to the next (quantum mottle) is the major limiting factor here due to the low counts used for image formation.

31c. True

The image is magnified, thus improving resolution; however, there is some geometrical distortion.

31d. False

Temporal indicates time; the output of light from the crystal lasts for a very small period of time, but during this period no further events will be detected (extra light output will merely be summed and probably excluded by the pulse height analyser [PHA]). This is known as dead time and leads to an underestimation of count rate.

31e. True

Bismuth germanate has a better detection efficiency at higher energy and so is used in PET where 511 keV gamma from positron annihilation is detected.

32a. True ****

The effective dose for a Tc-99 m bone scan is 5 mSv. For a barium enema it is 3–6 mSv.

32b. False

The effective dose for a thallium-201 cardiac scan is 18 mSv. Annual natural background radiation in the UK is 2–2.5 mSv.

32c. True

A Tc-99 m lung perfusion scan has an effective dose of 1 mSv, which is the same as the annual whole body dose limit for a member of the public.

32d. True

This removes radioactive urine from the bladder, reducing pelvic dose.

32e. False

Lead groin shields do not reduce the dose as the radiation source is internal.

33a. False ***

Although air in the syringe tip does need to be removed this should be done into a swab or container to prevent inhalation of airborne radionuclide and the risk of contamination.

33b. False

But these patients are usually kept away from general waiting areas and staff are advised to limit time spent in close contact.

33c. False

Radionuclides are usually bound to much larger pharmaceuticals; these can readily be removed with simple hand washing.

33d. True

Hospitals have limits for the activity they are allowed to release to the environment; gases can be vented, while solutions can be diluted and then released via the drains.

33e. False

It is acceptable to cordon off an area, wait until sufficient decay has occurred and then clean it up.

34a. True ****

The speed of sound in air is approximately 330 m/s, 1540 m/s in soft tissue, 3200 m/s in bone, and 4000 m/s in lead zirconate titanate (PZT).

34b. True

The speed of diagnostic ultrasound waves in soft tissue is relatively constant in all soft tissues and relatively independent of wavelength and frequency.

34c. False

Medical ultrasound waves can cause acceleration of particles up to 300 000 g and pressures of several atmospheres. Ultrasound can be used therapeutically to crack renal stones. Although it is largely considered safe at diagnostic levels, it should be kept in mind that ultrasound can cause cavitation, especially in antenatal scanning.

34d. False

Sound waves are longitudinal.

34e. True

Obviously it will take twice this length of time to receive an echo from an object 1 cm from the ultrasound probe.

35a. True ***

This means that the same element can both cause a wave via expansion when a voltage is applied, and can also create a voltage to be electronically read when a wave is received.

35b. False

The voltages used can be thousands of volts.

35c. False

Rapidly energising the transducers in a linear array sequentially from the periphery to the centre allows the beam to be focused to a set focal point. This is electronic focusing.

35d. False

The probe might typically transmit for 1 μs. It would then receive depending on the depth for maybe 200 μs for an object at approximately 15 cm depth. The receive time is dependent on the time for the ultrasound wave to travel from the probe to the maximum depth being scanned and back again.

35e. True

In a 3.5 MHz transducer abdominal probe this equates to an element approximately 0.5 mm thick.

36a. True ****

This refers to the size of the area of contact required with the patient. Since sector scanning fans out, the same area within the patient can be seen through a smaller window, or footprint.

36b. True

Speed of sound in soft tissue is relatively constant. To allow sound to travel further or deeper therefore with the same frame rate and scan line density, fewer pulses can be sent. There is always a compromise between these four features of realtime ultrasound imaging.

36c. False

Many contrast agents in ultrasound are merely microspheres of gas. This works because the difference in acoustic impedance between gas and tissue is large; sound is predominantly reflected, creating a high signal.

36d. True

This requires either computer controlled or monitored probe movement to allow correct orientation of slices.

36e. False

The first harmonic is the transmitted frequency. As sound travels through tissue it breaks down into its frequency components; numerically these are multiples of the transmitted frequency. The second harmonic is usually large enough to be detected and used for imaging; this can improve contrast, especially where there is a lot of tissue attenuation.

37a. True ****
This describes Doppler shift, the basis for the Doppler effect.

37b. True
The change in frequency is proportional to the object velocity:
Change in frequency/original frequency $= 2 \times$ (velocity of object/ velocity of sound)

37c. False
Doppler shift is at a maximum when the angle of insonation (angle between probe and moving object) is $0°$; at $90°$ no shift occurs.

37d. True
They usually range between 0 and 10 kHz. The audible sound range is 0.02–20 kHz

37e. True
Range gating is used to select areas for Doppler analysis.

38a. True *****
Also known as the z-axis. The individual proton dipoles do not point directly along the axis of the field but precess around it, in either a spin up or spin down state.

38b. False
Hydrogen nuclei (protons) in a uniform static magnetic field precess at the same frequency (Larmor frequency). This does vary ever so slightly depending on the substance the hydrogen is contained within, e.g. fat compared with water.

38c. False
1 T is approximately 25 000 times stronger than the earth's magnetic field.

38d. False
Larmor frequency (frequency of precession) is proportional to the magnetic field strength and the gyromagnetic ratio of the nucleus in question.

38e. False
An RF pulse has to equal the resonant/Larmor frequency in order to flip the magnetization vector. The flip angle is proportional to the strength and duration of the RF pulse.

39a. True ****
After the $90°$ pulse some proton spin vectors precess slightly more slowly and others slightly more quickly than the average Larmor frequency due to T2 relaxation processes and field inhomogeneities causing them to get out of phase. The NMR signal thus decays rapidly. A $180°$ pulse flips the vectors so that rather than moving out of phase the more quickly precessing vectors are now catching up with the slower vectors and they begin to rephase, producing a spin-echo at a later time, TE, after the initial $90°$ pulse. Only the dephasing effects of fixed field inhomogeneities are cancelled out, not the component due to true T2 relaxation. Thus a true T2-weighted signal is obtained.

39b. False
A GRE sequence does not cancel the dephasing effects of field inhomogeneities. The decay is T2* rather than a true T2.

39c. True

On some sequences a residual m_{xy} from the previous repetition would interfere with the next set of data obtained. To reduce this effect extra gradients or RF pulses can be introduced to 'spoil' and reduced to 0 the previous m_{xy} by dephasing it.

39d. True

The m_{xy} begins to dephase between the 90° and 180° pulses; it then needs an equal amount of time to rephase after being flipped by the 180° pulse until it returns to being in phase again; this is the echo.

39e. False

The GRE sequence is used when there is insufficient time for a 180° pulse to rephase the m_{xy}. As no rephasing occurs the echo is T2* and if the TE is long the echo will be of very small amplitude.

40a. False ***

A wider RF bandwidth will match the Larmor frequencies of a wider band of tissue if the field gradient remains the same; this will increase the thickness of slice selected.

40b. True

A steeper magnetic gradient will increase the range of Larmor frequencies of the body tissues. Thus a decreased thickness of tissue will have Larmor frequencies that lie within the RF bandwidth, and therefore a reduced thickness of slice will be selected.

40c. True

The steep phase encoding gradients produce the upper and lower lines of K-space, and the shallow phase encoding gradients produce the middle lines of K-space. The outer parts of K-space contribute most to the spatial resolution of the final image and the inner parts contribute most to the signal intensity of the image.

40d. False

The phase encoding gradient is switched on briefly at a time between slice selection and signal collection.

40e. True

Each sample of the recorded signal itself describes an 'echo' in 'pseudotime' as all phase encoding steps are played out. A 2D Fourier transform of K-space thus produces the final image.

T - #0584 - 101024 - C0 - 234/156/9 - PB - 9781853159510 - Gloss Lamination